Developing Nursing Knowledge

Philosophical Traditions and Influences

Developing Nursing Knowledge

Philosophical Traditions and Influences

BETH L. RODGERS, PhD, RN, FAAN

Professor
College of Nursing
University of Wisconsin-Milwaukee
Milwaukee, Wisconsin

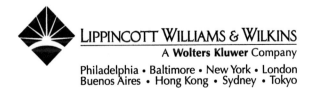

LIPPINCOTT WILLIAMS & WILKINS
A **Wolters Kluwer** Company
Philadelphia • Baltimore • New York • London
Buenos Aires • Hong Kong • Sydney • Tokyo

Acquisitions Editor: Margaret Zuccarini
Developmental Editor: Megan Klim
Editorial Assistant: Delema Caldwell-Jordan
Senior Production Editor: Rosanne Hallowell
Director of Nursing Production: Helen Ewan
Managing Editor / Production: Erika Kors
Design & Illustration Coordinator: Brett MacNaughton

Cover Designer: Melissa Walter
Interior Designer: Melissa Olson
Senior Manufacturing Manager: William Alberti
Indexer: Angie Wiley
Compositor: Lippincott Williams & Wilkins
Printer: R. R. Donnelley–Crawsfordsville

P2

Library of Congress Cataloging-in-Publication Data
Rodgers, Beth L.
   Developing nursing knowledge : philosophical traditions and influences / Beth L. Rodgers.
        p. ; cm.
     Includes index
     ISBN 0-7817-4708-2
   1. Nursing–Philosophy–History. 2.   Knowledge, Theory of–History. I. Title.
   [DNLM: 1.   Philosophy, Nursing–history. 2.   Knowledge. 3.   Nursing Theory. WY 11.1
R691d 2005]
RT84.5.R636 2005
610.73–dc22   2004014790

Care has been taken to confirm the accuracy of the information presented and to describe generally accepted practices. However, the author, editors, and publisher are not responsible for errors or omissions or for any consequences from application of the information in this book and make no warranty, express or implied, with respect to the content of the publication.

The author, editors, and publisher have exerted every effort to ensure that drug selection and dosage set forth in this text are in accordance with the current recommendations and practice at the time of publication. However, in view of ongoing research, changes in government regulations, and the constant flow of information relating to drug therapy and drug reactions, the reader is urged to check the package insert for each drug for any change in indications and dosage and for added warnings and precautions This is particularly important when the recommended agent is a new or infrequently employed drug.

Some drugs and medical devices presented in this publication have Food and Drug Administration (FDA) clearance for limited use in restricted research settings. It is the responsibility of the health care provider to ascertain the FDA status of each drug or device planned for use in his or her clinical practice.

LWW.com

To KVC and EBR,
My center;
It does hold.

REVIEWERS

KAREN LUCAS BREDA, PHD, MSN, RN
Associate Professor of Nursing
University of Hartford
West Hartford, Connecticut

MARION BROOME, PHD, RN, FAAN
Professor/Associate Dean for Research
University of Alabama at Birmingham
Birmingham, Alabama

SUSAN M. COHEN, DSN, APRN
Associate Professor
University of Pittsburgh
Pittsburgh, Pennsylvania

KAREN CROSBY, DNSC, RN, BC
Associate Professor
Brookdale Community College
Lincroft, New Jersey

JUDITH A. ERLEN, PHD, RN, FAAN
Professor and Doctoral Program
    Coordinator
University of Pittsburgh
Pittsburgh, Pennsylvania

AMY L. KENEFICK, PHD, RN, FNP
Assistant Professor
University of Connecticut
Storrs, Connecticut

MARJORIE MCINTYRE, RN, PHD
Associate Professor
University of Victoria
Victoria, British Columbia Canada

LINDA A. STREIT, RN, DSN, CCRN
Professor & Assistant Dean for the Graduate
    Program
Georgia Baptist College of Nursing of
    Mercer University
Atlanta, Georgia

PREFACE

Philosophy might seem like rather a rather odd area for nurses to explore. After all, nurses provide care, address clients' health needs, and draw on a knowledge base of complex pathophysiology, psychology, public health, management, leadership, politics, rehabilitation, and various other areas of knowledge that contribute to effective nursing. Where does philosophy fit into such a field?

The answer is: Everywhere. A nurse's thoughts and actions reflect nursing philosophy and the philosophy of the surrounding society. Philosophy influences important issues regarding truth, knowledge, inquiry, goodness, dignity, and health. As the nurse focuses on providing appropriate nursing care and conducting meaningful inquiry, it is easy to lose sight of how philosophy underlies everything that the nurse does—how the nurse sets goals, interacts with patients and families, shapes communities, influences the practice setting, and affects health policy. Taking the time and opportunity to explore how philosophy shapes these aspects of nursing will result in a much richer and fuller understanding of how nursing works, how it can be approached most effectively, and how it might be shaped to advance in the future.

One of the greatest skills that can be developed is the ability to critically analyze the positions of others and, in turn, to create one's own arguments. Merely to be able to recite what others have said, or to find the appropriate resources or references to justify a position is not adequate; limited to that level, learning is little more than the accumulation of the thoughts of others. Nursing, as well as the public at large, needs people who are able and willing to question, challenge, innovate, and create new and better ways of understanding the world and changing it for the better. Philosophy provides the basis and the skills for nurses to be active in shaping the future, not just anticipating it, preparing for it, or studying it once it is here.

There are many ways to embark on the study of philosophy as it pertains to nursing. Often, philosophy is presented thematically, such as examining together the writings on language, Truth, or aesthetics. For *Developing Nursing Knowledge: Philosophical Traditions and Influences,* I have chosen to use a more or less chronological progression, focusing on some of the major traditions that have helped to shape Western societies. I have chosen this format for several reasons. First, the chronological approach provides a sort of intellectual history, making it easier to see how philosophy has changed along certain lines of thought over the centuries. For example, in this arrangement it is evident how an early focus on knowledge turned to a focus on science in the 20th century and, later, evolved even further to emphasize human action and social structure as significant elements in the creation of knowledge. A chronology also demonstrates how philosophers do their work, engaging in what seems like an ongoing dialogue as they present their own views. Philosophers read, are influenced by, and often respond to the work of philosophers that preceded them. This type of dialogue sets a good example for nursing scholars by demonstrating the importance of discussion and debate to advance the discipline. *Developing Nursing Knowledge* provides an entry point to join in that dialogue. Finally, a chronologically oriented approach facilitates examining the various philosophies with reference to the context of the philosopher and the events and social situations associated with the period. Philosophers, like all humans, are influenced by the social contexts in which they develop their thoughts; understanding these contexts can provide important insights into the writer and the philosophical tradition. Reading the original works, of course, can add a much deeper dimension to the insights gained through this text.

An intellectual history approach has the limitation, however, of potentially giving the impression that the progression of ideas in philosophy is smooth and fluid. While there are some continuing threads and transitions, there is also a vast array of philosophical developments that have occurred through the ages that have influenced thought related to the development of nursing. The traditions and philosophers included in this text have been selected to provide a solid introduction to some of the most significant traditions relevant to nursing "science" and to promote philosophical thinking as a means to develop skills of critique and argumentation. Perhaps most importantly, this text is intended to facilitate development of the desire and the skills to question the thinking of others and the ideology that surrounds us every day, and to learn to question our own thinking just as well.

By creating this text, I have hoped to point out some of the big questions that exist for nurses in regard to our knowledge base, and how just a few influential philosophers, in their widely varying ways, have attempted to answer those questions. In doing so, I hope it is clear just how many ways there are to look at the world and to look at nursing. More than anything, I hope to promote a spirit of inquiry, questioning, creativity, and innovation.

In preparing this text, it has been necessary to make some decisions about what traditions and philosophers to include and what could, perhaps, wait for another time. The intent in *Developing Nursing Knowledge*—to generate curiosity as well as some introductory level of familiarity with Western philosophy—has made the selection of traditions fairly simple. I included the philosophers that have been of most widespread influence and familiarity in our field. The reader of this text should have sufficient background to converse with others about some of the major issues concerning science and knowledge development. Unfortunately, that selection meant excluding some of the philosophies that could influence nursing. Particularly intriguing in this regard are the Chinese and Indian philosophies, which are rich in their similarity to the views of humans and health espoused in nursing. Yet even these philosophies are best considered in juxtaposition to the prevailing epistemology and philosophy of science under which we experience much of our education in the West. As a result, *Developing Nursing Knowledge: Philosophical Traditions and Influences* should be considered the departure point for a journey through philosophy as it has, and might, influence us as nurses.

I am fortunate to have had the opportunity to share just such a journey with many wonderful students over the years. I hope some of them, along with others who read this text, will someday become colleagues who enjoy exploring the nature and development of our knowledge base. I applaud their inquisitiveness, their challenging questions, and their high ideals. This book is for them, and for anyone else who believes that, by being thorough in our reflection and by learning to look at things in a different way, we can achieve much greater potential as nurses and as humans as we assume our small place in this complex world. I am grateful to the outstanding staff at Lippincott Williams & Wilkins for taking on this project with me, for understanding the need for nurses to explore philosophy, and for their support and assistance throughout the preparation of this text. I am also forever indebted to Dr. Kathleen Cowles who provided invaluable editorial assistance, tangible and moral support, gentle prodding, and always a burst of humor when it was most needed.

Beth L. Rodgers, PhD, RN, FAAN

CONTENTS

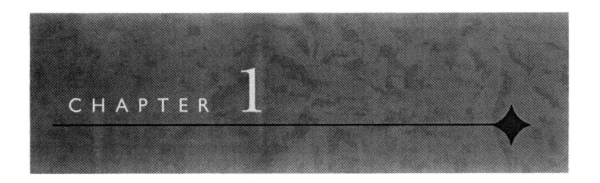

CHAPTER 1

Understanding Nursing Knowledge

KEY IDEAS

borrowing of knowledge   nursing perspective
discipline   paradigm
epistemology   science
knowledge

Nurses often find themselves in situations where they need to answer the important question "what do nurses do?" Clinicians, administrators, researchers, and other nursing scholars have argued for decades that the ability to describe the work of nurses will provide the public and other disciplines with a greater understanding of the nature of nursing and nursing practice. There is no clear and simple answer to this question; however, it is difficult to formulate a response that effectively captures the work of nurses. What nurses *do* might be described by citing a list of activities such as assess health status, administer medications, teach, provide psychosocial support, intervene with families, prepare patients for discharge, make referrals. Taxonomies have been developed that reflect these types of interventions and provide a basis for research and measurement of outcomes (Coenen, Ryan, & Sutton, 1997; Elasy, Ellis, Brown, & Pichert, 2001; Henry, Holzemer, & Miller, 1997; Moorhead & Delaney, 1997; Thoroddsen & Thorsteinssen, 2002). The general public and other non-nurses would probably understand these activities without difficulty. Most nurses would have a number of items to add to the list; however, much of what nurses find to be most important in their work involves activities that are not easily understood by non-nurses. Actions such as "being there" for someone (Steeves, Cohen, & Wise, 1994), "being present" (Gilje, 1992), "therapeutic use of self" (Cumbie, 2001; Gallop & O'Brien, 2003; Sherman & Ouelette, 2001; Uys, 1980), "empathic understanding" (Ruffing-Rahal, 1986), "promoting expanding consciousness" (Newman, 1986), "caring for the whole person," or simply "caring" (Watson, 1979, 1988; Watson & Smith, 2002) comprise much of the work of nursing and may actually capture some of its greatest value.

In spite of the value of such a description, there is a far more important underlying component of nursing that needs attention. What makes nurses valuable is not just what they do; it is the **knowledge** supporting their actions that distinguishes nurses from other providers and the lay public. The most important question for nurses to address really concerns not what they *do*, but what they *know*.

Understanding and being able to describe what nurses know requires more than merely the ability to list areas of content covered in educational programs. Discussion of the knowledge base of nursing also requires more than the ability to describe how the nurse makes decisions on a daily basis. Nurses need to be able to question their own knowledge, identify assumptions and biases, and recognize alternative ways of thinking in various situations. Nurses also need to be critical and insightful about their knowledge base to promote continuing development and recognize areas for further inquiry. An understanding of some of the major traditions in philosophy is essential in this process of knowing and developing the knowledge of nurses.

THE NATURE OF NURSING KNOWLEDGE

Nurse researchers and scholars have given comparatively little attention to the question of nursing *knowledge*. Similarly, nurses in practice settings are not accustomed to discussing the nature of their knowledge, such as how and what they know; instead they discuss only *that* they know something and that they can do something as a result. In an acute care setting, for example, a nurse may "know" to position emergency equipment near a patient's room, feeling quite certain that it will be needed to care for the patient in the near future. The nurse may "know" that sitting quietly with a patient, just "being there," has a therapeutic effect. If so inclined, the nurse may touch the patient in a way that is expected to transfer energy to the depleted individual. If asked how the nurse "knows" to do these things, the answer often would be limited to "I just know."

To describe their roles, nurse clinicians need to formulate useful descriptions and understandings of nursing that focus on the knowledge they possess. Awareness of the knowledge base not only captures the special education and experiences associated with being a nurse but also serves as the foundation for accountability for the care the nurse provides. The rationale "I just know" does not provide the nurse with much security that any actions taken are appropriate and defensible. However, an emphasis on what nurses know combined with how they know these things provides a basis not only for accountability for actions but also for explaining to others their significant contributions to health care.

Understanding the origins and foundations of nursing knowledge serves yet another purpose. Many of the things nurses value and the tasks they perform on a regular basis are not understood well by nurses or by other health care professionals, nor has research shown these actions to be effective or appropriate. For example, nurses often describe the important role that intuition plays in clinical practice (Agan, 1987; Kenny, 1994; King & Appleton, 1997; Paley, 1996; Sarvimäki & Stenbock-Hult, 1996), and those who have studied therapeutic or healing touch (Begley, 2002; Daley, 1997; Meehan, 1998; Peters, 1999; Thomas, 2002; Turner, Clark, & Williams, 1998; Wright, 1987; Yamashita, Jensen, & Tall, 1998) or essential oils may use these techniques as healing agents or as an adjunct to their usual care. Nurses address the human spirit as an essential focus of care (Lawson & Horneffer, 2002), even though it may be difficult to define this "spirit." Nurses base much of their practice and their skill on the premise that humans are holistic, "biopsychosocial" beings (Flaskerud & Halloran, 1980; Kim, 1987). How do nurses know these things? Doing, teaching, learning, and caring all require knowledge; to continue to grow and improve in these areas, it is essential to understand how the knowledge needed by nurses can be created.

Nurses in practice settings are not the only ones who need to be concerned with the knowledge base of the discipline and the means to develop knowledge. Researchers must be attentive to issues surrounding knowledge by performing their investigations with the primary purpose of enhancing nursing's knowledge base. As a result, they must be keenly aware of issues related to knowledge and the implications of various viewpoints on the methods used for knowledge development. Without such attention, researchers may use inappropriate methodologies, or use methodologies inappropriately, and be limited in their ability to justify their work to the nursing and scientific communities. The history of nursing contains numerous examples where lack of consideration of philosophical issues concerning knowledge has limited the scope of problems addressed and the methodologies used to enhance the nursing knowledge base. The emphasis on knowledge generation inherent in research requires that scholars have an in-depth awareness of what it *means* to generate knowledge.

THE HISTORY OF NURSING KNOWLEDGE

Certainly nurses have not been functioning without the benefit of substantive knowledge. Many authors and scholars in the past, however, have argued that much of this knowledge was not truly "nursing knowledge." Instead a number of leaders in nursing have argued that the knowledge used by nurses was "borrowed" from other disciplines (Feldman, 1981; Johnson, 1968; Visintainer, 1986). Nurses do use information created in other fields in many ways. For example, psychology provides an essential basis for nurses to understand the stress and coping responses of people experiencing illness and life changes. Nurses did not discover nor did they create much of the knowledge concerning physiology, medical treatment, pharmacology, and infection control that underlies a great deal of nursing care.

Nursing Education

The history of nursing supports this contention about nursing knowledge and the borrowing of knowledge from other disciplines to some extent. Organized nursing is a relatively recent development, emerging from nursing's early foundation in lay caregiving and in the religious orders focused on assisting the infirm. Religious orders, in response to the need of the ill for care and assistance, developed the early institutions that resembled the hospitals of today. Duty and responsibility motivated the lay family caregiver, while in religious settings a sense of beneficence and altruism led groups of monks and nuns to provide care for those in need. Over time, a variety of social, economic, and political circumstances in Europe and in America led health care away from those beneficent roots. By the 17th and 18th centuries, the majority of hospitals in America and Europe presented abominable conditions for care. Few physicians had formal medical education, and the most undesirable members of society performed the work of "nurses." People with all types of criminal and abusive vices gradually replaced religious providers as the primary providers of service for the ill and infirm.

While Florence Nightingale promoted major reforms of nursing and especially schools and training for nurses, no formal education for nurses existed before the Nightingale reform movement. The earliest efforts at developing "education" for nurses provided some basic preparation but still fell far short of the educational standards of modern times. Early programs primarily focused on the careful selection of young women who would become nurses. School administrators particularly sought young women of character and "plain looks." Such personal characteristics typically took precedence over any concern for the content of the schooling; some of the early inquiry done in nursing continued to address the characteristics most appropriate for a good nurse. Nursing education was referred to as "training," a term that persisted within the vernacular of nursing; these training programs followed primarily an apprenticeship model. Gradually it became obvious that nurses needed some formal education, particularly in the areas of biology and anatomy. In the mid- to late 1800s in America, physicians primarily provided the didactic content. Nurses learned the actual skills of "nursing" through on-the-job experiences.

Nursing schools slowly proliferated through the West as the need for nurses grew and emphasis on the importance of "training" increased. These schools were associated with hospitals rather than academic settings, and served as much to provide a work force for the hospitals as they did to train nurses. Structured content provided to nurses almost exclusively came from medicine and the natural sciences, while the substantive work of nursing was learned by "doing." Schools were, in fact, commonly discouraged from expanding nursing content; nursing was regarded by many as a noble "calling." In an article in the *New York Medical Journal*, physician W. Gilman Thompson (1908) argued that nursing clearly was not a profession because nurses did not have the specialized knowledge befitting a professional. Instead, he saw nursing as a calling, and indicated that any woman could easily learn how to obey the instructions of physicians. Schools for nurses did not become a part of academic settings until well into the 20th century in the United States, as nursing moved away from the status of vocational only. Decades passed before instructors in these programs had been educated in academically oriented programs of nursing.

A similar situation existed in regard to graduate level education for nurses. Although Master's level preparation in nursing was established in the early 1930s, development of programs at this level proceeded very slowly. Although there were programs for nurses to achieve doctoral degrees, real growth in this movement was not evident until the 1960s. The earliest programs were associated with existing programs in the discipline of education. Thus nurses with early doctoral education tended to have been socialized in the ways of education. To promote the development of more nurses with doctoral level education for purposes of teaching and biomedical research, many nurse scholars and leaders achieved degrees in other fields often under the auspices of the Nurse Scientist Program developed by the United States Public Health Service for this purpose. It is only since the 1970s and early 1980s that the people responsible for the education of nurses have been educated within nursing and from what might be called a "nursing perspective."

Shared Knowledge

In reality, nurses had been sharing knowledge throughout history through their various training programs and as colleagues and mentors. The "on-the-job" learning certainly involved sharing experience and personal insights gained through years of providing diligent care. The work of nursing and the knowledge that provided its foundation were not studied or documented; still this essential learning was handed down across generations of nurses through their interactions.

This form of knowledge has been critical to the development of nursing and to its current practice. Preceptorships, practica, and other forms of experiential learning provide not only the opportunity for students to practice what they have learned through classroom and other didactic components of their educational programs but also to learn through a mentoring and experiential model. This model forms a sort of "oral tradition" in nursing that is essential to professional socialization and the provision of optimal patient care. However, this type of learning lacks the structure and other qualities that enable it to be recognized as legitimate and valuable, particularly in comparison to the model of "science." The latter science model has been the benchmark for knowledge throughout modern times in Western societies and continues to place demands on the development of nursing as a discipline and a profession.

Borrowed Knowledge

Many writers in the discipline have viewed the lack of "nursing" emphasis in the nursing knowledge base as quite troublesome in the earlier stages of nursing knowledge development. Problems associated with the **"borrowing" of knowledge** include the possible pitfalls of directly applying knowledge developed in other disciplines that presumably was developed for other purposes or needs. Some authors argued that such knowledge would have to be altered to conform to a **nursing perspective** or at minimum tested and validated to ensure its appropriateness within a nursing context (Hardy, 1978; Johnson, 1968). Concepts and meanings do change across contexts, and knowledge created in other fields or for other purposes may work differently when used in new or unique ways.

Another significant concern has revolved around the specific needs of nurses and the unique phenomena they confront in their various roles. If nurses rely on other disciplines to generate the knowledge they need, there is considerable risk that important questions in nursing will not be addressed. Because of their particular viewpoint on health and illness, nurses often see problems that are passed over by persons in other disciplines or that may be addressed in ways inappropriate for use by nurses. A physiologist, for example, will see mobility problems in an older adult from the standpoint of the body's structure and function and the various physical factors that affect human kinetics. The nurse, however, will recognize that while physical structure and function are important, investigation into an individual's motivation and attitude along with assessment and possible alteration in the environment can do wonders to improve mobility. If the inquiry is left to others, issues associated with environmental change regarding mobility may not be addressed at all or certainly not to the extent needed by nurses.

A substantial body of knowledge has been created that supports the work of nursing and the development of the discipline. The *Annual Review of Nursing Research* has been published for nearly 2 decades and provides a comprehensive synthesis of nursing research addressing a wide range of phenomena. Taxonomies useful in capturing the nature of nursing work and related outcomes (Johnson, Maas, & Moorhead, 2000; McCloskey & Bulechek, 2000) have been in continuing development for a long time as well. These activities are evidence of the important work of nurses and accelerating progress in developing the discipline's knowledge base. Inquiry and knowledge development must continue; however, this work must be flexible in meeting the changing needs of the discipline as well as the dynamic contexts and multiple realms in which nurses work and conduct research.

Nursing often seems to fall short of the ideals of "science" in evaluation of the knowledge base. Consequently nurses may refer to other essential components of the knowledge base as representing the "art" of nursing. Discussion of nursing

> **BOX I-I**
>
> ## IMPORTANCE OF NURSING KNOWLEDGE DEVELOPMENT
>
> ◆ Articulate knowledge base of nurses rather than tasks.
> ◆ Address problems relevant to nurses.
> ◆ Take responsibility for continuing development of the discipline.
> ◆ Approach inquiry from a perspective of nursing.

knowledge, however, lacks review and evaluation of that standard of "science," determination of its legitimacy, and consideration of other valid ways of developing knowledge. Only a philosophical examination of "science" and of "knowledge" in general can provide nurses with the foundation needed to appropriately evaluate and develop nursing's knowledge base. The use of knowledge from other fields might solve part of the problem of "science." Such an approach, however, poses risks from the standpoint of the need to ensure that the whole of knowledge is understood. Taking just a piece of knowledge without regard to the original framework could result in the knowledge being fragmented. This, in turn, would open the user to possible significant errors in interpretation.

These are cautions, however, that need to be considered with all knowledge. To ensure that they employ the best practices possible, nurses must be able to take advantage of all the information available to them. Over-reliance on borrowed knowledge, however, enables nurses to deflect the responsibility for solving problems onto researchers in other fields. The only way to be certain that the problems and knowledge needs of nurses are met is for nurses to have an active role in the discovery or development of the knowledge. While there is great deal of essential or useful knowledge available for nurses, researchers in other fields have not addressed adequately many areas of practice for which nurses need a solid knowledge base (Box 1-1).

So far, it is clear that nurses do use knowledge developed in other fields but they also have developed and need to further develop knowledge specific to their own foci and problems within practice and the discipline. Nurses need to be able to describe, justify, and defend what nurses *know* and how they can be assured in their knowledge claims. Finally to determine the most appropriate and effective directions for future inquiry, there is a need to consider the disparate ways in which knowledge can be developed. Nursing is far too advanced at present to continue to explain its level of development as embryonic, or emerging, or pre-paradigmatic and to rely on other dogmatic statements about nursing as "art and science" without being able to explain these distinctions. The observation that some elements of nursing do not seem to meet traditional standards of "science" should not evoke "art" as an explanation for the seemingly non-science component as if these two ideas constitute a dichotomous explanation of knowledge. Instead such an observation should prompt the nurse to reexamine the standard of science. It is quite likely that on close examination many of the statements regarded as self-evident in nursing will be found to be hindrances rather than facilitators of growth and progress (Rodgers, 1991).

 # KNOWLEDGE DEVELOPMENT

Nursing as a Discipline

In efforts to stimulate development of the knowledge base of nursing, many writers and leaders in the field described guidelines or foci that could give direction to development of the discipline. One aspect of such discussion placed emphasis on the nature of a *discipline*, in the apparent belief that awareness of what constituted a discipline would provide the understanding needed to guide the development of nursing as a discipline. Donaldson and Crowley (1978) produced a widely read article on the nature of the discipline of nursing, pointing out the need for identification of "the essence of nursing research and of the common elements and threads that give coherence to an identifiable body of knowledge" (p. 113). Arguing that much of the foundation for nursing was "tacit rather than explicit" (p. 113), they encouraged effort to clarify the nature of the discipline of nursing to ensure that research in nursing was, indeed, *nursing* research rather than nurses merely doing research appropriate to *other* disciplines. Their approach to the dilemma concerning the nature of the discipline of nursing was to draw on discussions of disciplinary structure, such as those presented by Schwab (1964a, 1964b) and Shermis (1962), as a means to provide clear direction for future developments.

According to Schwab (1964a, 1964b) along with other scholars of his genre and as supported initially in nursing by Donaldson and Crowley (1978), a **discipline** is characterized by a substantive structure and a syntax. The substantive structure of a discipline is the content, in other words, the conceptualizations, theories, principles, etc. that determine the focus of interest and the scope of inquiry. The syntax involves the methodologies and the means to determine the appropriateness or credibility of knowledge developed within the discipline. Both of these occur within a broader perspective that characterizes the discipline.

Carper (1975) tried a different approach by identifying the types of knowledge that characterize nursing. Through "systematic analysis of selected nursing literature" (abstract), Carper identified four types of knowledge used in nursing: empirics, esthetics, personal knowledge, and ethics. These patterns of knowing were considered to represent an important part of the structure of the discipline. Carper's work (1978) left a memorable mark on theoretical discussion of nursing by showing the complexity of the discipline. A focus on types of knowledge also revealed the inappropriateness of categorizations of nursing based on medical constructions or disease terminology. Carper proposed that "nursing process" was "the primary method of inquiry in the field of nursing" (p. 108), thus serving as an important component of the syntax of the discipline.

Other authors approached the idea of the nature of the discipline of nursing from the standpoint of nursing's uniqueness. The distinction between basic and applied sciences was a common element of such discussions (Donaldson & Crowley, 1978; Johnson, 1959) and authors frequently pointed out that nursing was a "practice" or "professional" discipline and, thus, had distinct needs and purposes that set it apart from more traditional (i.e., basic) scientific disciplines (for example, physics or chemistry). Dickoff's and James' (1968) discussion of types of theory was consistent with this emphasis because they identified different types or levels of theory relative to purpose and stage of development of the knowledge base. The fourth and highest level of theory was referred to as "situation-producing" theory and was identified as the type most appropriate for theory development in nursing (Dickoff & James, 1968).

Theory Development

In the late 1960s in an effort to promote systematic expansion of knowledge appropriate for nursing and to explore mechanisms for elevating the status of nursing within scientific communities, noted nurse leaders and scholars began to focus on the discipline's substantive structure as a means to promote development of nursing (Flaskerud & Halloran, 1980; Kim, 1987). Many writers in this era placed a primary emphasis on the development of theory in the belief that the substantive content of the discipline needed to be nursing-specific theoretical formulations. Indeed a number of philosophers of science had focused on theory as the product of "science" (Ayer, 1959; Hempel, 1952; Kuhn, 1962; Popper, 1972). For the substance of nursing to be a **science**, nurse scholars would need to develop clear theories that were relevant to practice and consistent with the goals and perspective of the discipline (Nursing Theories Conference Group, 1980). Beginning with the 1960s and continuing well into the 1980s, this emphasis on theory development was a prominent theme in nursing for more than 20 years.

Several factors contributed to a flurry of activity during this time. As previously discussed, one obvious force was the idea of "uniqueness," and the belief that development of theory in nursing would ensure a continuing position for nurses in health care delivery. In addition to ensuring viability, nurses sought a higher status as "professionals." Earlier studies in sociology (Dingwall & Lewis, 1983) had led to the belief that a unique knowledge base was an essential characteristic of a profession. Consistent with this position, many nurse leaders argued that without the ability to delineate their knowledge and unique contributions, nurses could not achieve the status they desired as "professionals;" they would be seen as merely "staff" much like a laborer position in health care institutions.

The growing affiliation of graduate level programs in university settings also created a situation wherein nursing needed to conform to an academic model. Prevailing ideology based on philosophical trends in academic disciplines of the time led nurses in two directions in their knowledge development foci. First nurses needed to develop not just knowledge but also "science." Throughout modern times, science has been viewed as the highest, most rigorous form of knowledge. For nursing to compete with other disciplines, especially medicine and other established fields, nurses needed to be able to articulate that their practice was based on a credible foundation of "science." In an effort to determine means to develop this science, scholars turned to the philosophy of science for direction as to what constitutes science and credible scientific methodologies. Here they found their second imperative for the development of nursing. According to prevailing ideology at the time, a defining characteristic of "science" was the existence of well defined "theory." Heeding the words of prominent 20th century philosophers of science, nurses recognized that all these contemporary philosophers of science had a primary focus on theory as the product of scientific activity despite their diverse positions. This emphasis on theory development was reflected in a highly popular book in nursing at the time (Reynolds, 1971). Reynolds' text is referenced extensively in the writings of nurse scholars and theorists during this time; this shows the influence of these ideas at this point in nursing's history. Thus the race was on to develop a theory base for nursing.

A wide variety of theories was created during the time of this emphasis on theory development to provide the substantive foundation for the discipline. Numerous books provide details of the theories, and critiques of this movement and the theoretical products are abundant (Fawcett, 1988; Frederickson, 1993; Fitzpatrick, 1987, 1988; Murphy & Schmitz, 1979; Rawls, 1980). Exploring these theories in detail is not this text's purpose. More importantly, this general overview considers the various events that occurred in the context of developing the knowledge base for nursing and recognizes theory's role and emphasis as a part of the discipline's evolution.

During this significant part of nursing's history, nurse leaders sought a substantive foundation for nursing through the development of "theory." They presumed the presence of a clearly delineated theory base would meet nursing's needs in a number of ways. The "nursing theory" would satisfy the demand for a unique knowledge base, providing evidence of what nurses do and ensuring their place in health care. Similarly developing nursing theory would promote the position of nursing schools in academic settings by demonstrating not only the unique knowledge base but more importantly that nursing constitutes a "science."

The theory movement in nursing marks the beginning of an enduring focus in nursing on articulating and developing the knowledge base of the discipline. Discussions surrounding theory have been fraught with references to philosophy and the direction it provided as to what constituted theory, what makes a "good" theory, and appropriate methodologies for developing theory. Many schools of nursing selected a specific theory as the organizing framework for their curricula, and some health care institutions have taken similar steps to incorporate the identified theories in their philosophy and mission statements. Several of the theories continue to be used, tested, and developed, and disseminated widely several decades after their initial development (Fitzpatrick, 1988; Frederickson, 1993; Johnson, 1980; King, 1971, 1981; Levine, 1966; Murphy & Schmitz, 1979; Neuman, 1972, 1986; Orem, 1971; Orlando, 1961; Parker, 1991; Parse, 1981; 1980; Rogers, 1970; Roy, 1970, 1971; Watson, 1979; Yamashita, Jensen, & 1998).

After the initial flurry of activity and widespread acceptance of this theory development focus, there was a waning of attention to these theories; in fact, overt rejection of this movement and the exclusive focus on nurse-developed theories is evident in the discipline in the years that followed. Perhaps too high an expectation had been placed on these products and they fell short of meeting the desire for presenting all-encompassing descriptions of nurses' work and thinking. They have been criticized for their lack of specificity needed to direct nursing practice; some contained esoteric terminology that made them difficult to use in communicating the role of nurses in public and interdisciplinary forums. Most were developed deductively through logic, reasoning, and reflection rather than through testing in practice situations; so their linkages to practice were strained in many cases. The lack of validation through "scientific" testing also placed these "theories" at odds with the prevailing philosophy that stimulated their development. The phrase "theoretical framework" or "conceptual framework," rather than the word "theory," often was used to describe these constructions. That nurses had sought complete, finished products, that is, a final answer to the question "What is Nursing?" also worked against these theoretical developments; there initially was a lack of effort to develop them further to enhance their usefulness to the discipline.

The last several decades, while an exciting and provocative phase in nursing knowledge development, also were tumultuous. The number of nurses with advanced education in nursing has increased exponentially, whereas previously doctoral education had been obtained in other fields. This has contributed to the emergence of new perspectives on nursing knowledge rather than continuing transfer of other disciplines' ways to nursing. Nurses also have attended more closely to changes in philosophy; this has provided alternate ways of thinking about disciplines and about science and knowledge in general.

During this time, philosophy and ideas about what constitutes "science" have changed as well. Kuhn (1962) introduced the concept of "paradigm" as a hallmark of science; he argued that a science was distinguished by the fact that scientists in a discipline worked within the frame of reference provided by the prevailing "paradigm"; the presence of *theory* did not distinguish a science. According to Kuhn, the **paradigm** functioned as a "disciplinary matrix" and contained the concepts and rules appropriate to the intellectual work of the members of the discipline. While theory still was viewed as the end product of scientific activity, Kuhn presented a case whereby there was reason to believe that explication of nursing's "paradigm" would distinguish nursing as a unique discipline and, at least of equal importance, as a science. The rather broad ideas and theories that previously had characterized the substance of nursing were reconsidered in light of their representations of nursing's "paradigm." There was consistency among the existing theories in the reliance on the fundamental concepts of nursing, health, environment, and "man" (more recently addressed as "person"), and a consensus resulted that these were the primary concepts of interest in nursing. The theories typically addressed nursing in a very general sense as assisting people in both health and illness situations to grow and develop as whole persons, achieving higher states of development and well-being to the extent possible. Despite the debate regarding the position and purpose of the nursing theories, this effort contributed significantly to generating consensus on the overall orientation of nursing and its philosophy and values. More recently, their value as theories has increased particularly as philosophy has altered its approach to what may appropriately be called "theory."

Throughout this time it is clear that nursing was attempting to follow the direction set by philosophy of science to steer its development and knowledge building activities. Often what was considered to be the knowledge base of the discipline fell short of the standards set in philosophy. Nurses could not find appropriate or acceptable ways to do research on what was called "intuition," which nurses relied on in their daily practices or to explore aspects of spirituality, an important component of nursing care. Traditional scientific methods also did not fit other significant aspects of nursing such as empathy or "presence" or rising interest in alternative care modalities. Similarly, whatever knowledge might be available or created to help nurses determine what to do in a situation, it would not necessarily describe *how* the nurse should act or account for the specific actions of nurses. In other words, knowledge might help nurses to think and decide what to do, but it would not necessarily tell them how to be skillful at carrying out those actions. Because of the limitations of the extant view of "science," scholars in nursing tended to differentiate nursing as both science and "art," where "art" was used to capture aspects of nursing that did not fit the traditional mold of "science."

NURSING KNOWLEDGE AS A FOUNDATION FOR NURSING PRACTICE AND RESEARCH

Nurses continue to recognize their field as both an "art" and a "science" (Rodgers, 1991; Rogers, 1988; Smith, 1997; Watson, 1994). Such a characterization accomplishes several things. First, it provides a way of describing the knowledge that underlies nursing practice. It accounts for many important aspects of nursing that do not fit the mold of "science." Finally as with any characterization, it promotes some cohesion within the discipline as nurses share this perception and a common way to describe their work.

But it raises a number of questions as well. Is there not knowledge behind the art? How do nurses validate that knowledge? How can research be conducted concerning that art? How can it be taught? How can nurses be held accountable in the use of that "art" in interactions with patients? The ability to demonstrate outcomes for that art and to justify the essential work of nurses in their contributions to health care is particularly important in an economic context and for nursing's own evaluation and growth.

The Role of Philosophy: Understanding Nursing Knowledge

Rather than launch into in-depth study of art, it is most prudent to step back and take a broader look at the entire realm of nursing knowledge. The distinction of art and science arose from a philosophy that has long been supplanted by new ideas about science and knowledge. While art and aesthetics have a great deal to offer nurses, continuing to dwell on this dichotomy can only perpetuate some of the weaknesses in this description of nursing. It is counterproductive as well in that many of the things that would fall under the heading of "art" are the things that nurses tend to value most. Yet the surrounding culture demands a "science" approach to knowledge. Philosophy offers a wide array of viewpoints and arguments from which nurses can re-evaluate the knowledge base of nursing and perhaps construct even stronger and more useful characterizations. This calls for an examination of not just nursing "science," but a look at the broader realm of "nursing knowledge." Understanding what constitutes knowledge, how knowledge can be created and validated, and the many types of available knowledge provides nurses with the background and skill necessary to continue to develop the foundations for quality nursing practice and for the growth of the discipline. Most important, this understanding allows nurses to set their own directions for knowledge rather than follow the lead of academic initiatives and other disciplines that bear little resemblance to nursing.

The nature of knowledge is the focus of a particular branch of philosophy referred to as **epistemology**. Epistemology is, by definition, the study of knowledge. From a general standpoint, **knowledge** is defined as justified, true belief. It involves a number of facets, for example:

Under what conditions can we consider something to be "knowledge"?
When is it appropriate to say "I know..."?
What are we really saying when we use the phrase "I know..."?
How is knowledge differentiated from habit, custom, intuition, opinion, or belief?
Do different types or forms of knowledge exist?
What are the means for validation or justification of knowledge?
What constitutes "truth"?

For a statement to count as an element of knowledge, the statement or facts must be justified using philosophically defensible means: it must be "true" and there should be some degree of "certainty" according to most views. In other words, the nurse should be able to count on the information to be a reliable or accurate reflection of the situation.

All these terms—justification, defensible, true, certain—are critical to the discussion of knowledge and to the development of the knowledge base for the discipline of nursing. Immediately a conceptual problem is apparent, that is, these terms can all be defined in many different ways. The particular definition employed will have a profound effect on the strategies used to develop and justify the knowledge base of nursing. It is not just a matter of the nurse being able to say with some degree of comfort "I know" but also being able to have faith in that statement and to defend it to others who may not have that knowledge.

Knowledge and Science

At this point, an understanding of philosophy is critical. The questions identified so far in this discussion are just a few generated by the study of knowledge. To date, nurses have answered these questions from the standpoint of what is regarded as traditional science, exemplified by data collection, description, and experimentation. Many of these questions of interest to nurses have been answered quite inadequately from the standpoint of the discipline of nursing. Science does not enable nurses to say "I know" about many of the things of interest to them. With an understanding of philosophy and the many possible approaches to knowledge development, it becomes clear that "science" may not be the only way to create a substantive foundation for the work of nurses. Perhaps science should be redefined so that areas of interest to nurses can be admitted as science. Perhaps alternatives to science are available that enable nurses to have faith in their knowledge even if some may not look like traditional science. The study of philosophy can provide the material and arguments needed to formulate an appropriate and defensible means for nursing to progress through rigorous inquiry.

In addition, philosophy has changed since nursing adopted many of the early dominant conceptions of knowledge and science. There are a variety of ways to view knowledge and approaches to its development that may be legitimized for purposes of advancing the discipline of nursing. The challenge is not to succumb to any particular dominant approach but to be able to make reasoned and defensible arguments for progress in the discipline. There is no single, timeless, "right" answer for questions concerning nursing's knowledge base and the nature of the discipline. Arguments, some of which are defensible and some of which are far less convincing, can be presented about all these important issues.

 CONCLUSION

The study of philosophy can be immensely helpful in this endeavor because the study of knowledge and science, what counts as these and how they are created, is one of the primary interests of philosophers It is possible that there are other ways to view the discipline and justify the work of nurses without relying on traditional forms of research and views of "science." A broad look at the many ways in which knowledge is constituted is needed for nursing to advance. The search for options and alternate ways to create, support, and understand knowledge can provide nurses with the direction needed to promote progress in the discipline.

Nurses also need to be able to think philosophically about their knowledge base and make sound judgments about its continuing development. Understanding philosophy and its contributions and influence on the nature of knowledge is not an easy task. Without some understanding, however, nurses are placed in the precarious position of blindly following the lead of other disciplines, whose needs and foci may not be relevant to the work of nurses and their knowledge base. Perhaps even more detrimental, a potential outcome is the fact that nurses may attempt to formulate arguments for their work and knowledge without the benefit of the centuries of effort devoted to this topic by philosophers and other scholars. Without such understanding, nurses can scarcely comprehend the evolution of their own discipline and profession because its development has been subject to the influences of philosophy of which they may or may not be aware. Viewed in the context of its own time and in the context of nursing history, philosophy provides the very foundation for nursing knowledge.

Since the beginning of recorded history (and possibly before), humans have sought to understand the world around them and to have some mastery and sense of certainty about how the world works and how it may unfold. The questions that confront nurse theorists, researchers, and scholars have puzzled humans since the beginning of thought. Unfortunately most of what is learned about knowledge is limited to traditional methods of science as it has been conducted in modern times (that is, for most of the last two centuries). Yet it has not always been envisioned in such a way. An examination of major thoughts and movements in Western intellectual history provides insights into the many ways in which knowledge has been viewed, the merits and limitations of these viewpoints, and alternate ways of considering and developing the knowledge base of nursing. Solid research skills are one prerequisite for development of the knowledge base for nursing; understanding of philosophy and what makes those skills "solid" is another crucial part of the process.

The journey in the ensuing pages is one of exploration and enlightenment. The focus is not on finding the answers to what puzzles nurses in their efforts to create and expand the knowledge base. Indeed it is questionable that even the relevant problems are clear. Effort first must be directed toward expanding the perspective and becoming aware of the many ways in which knowledge can be viewed and developed. The foundations to be explored are not the answers and substantive knowledge, but the foundation that philosophy, with its questioning and controversy and inquisitiveness, provides for the growth of nursing knowledge.

FOR DISCUSSION

1. Identify and analyze examples of statements about nursing that are considered to be self-evident and that shape thinking and development in the discipline (nursing dogma).
2. Discuss ways in which knowledge is shared among disciplines. Give examples of nursing knowledge that might be used in other disciplines.
3. Explore the relationships that exist in the knowledge base of nursing and other related disciplines.
4. Identify elements of nursing that make it a unique discipline. What elements make it less unique?
5. Discuss possible answers to the question "What do nurses know?"

REFERENCES

Agan, R. D. (1987). Intuitive knowing as a dimension of nursing. *Advances in Nursing Science, 10*(1), 63–70.

Ayer, A. J. (Ed.). (1959). *Logical positivism*. Glencoe, IL: Free Press.

Begley, S. S. (2002). The energetic language of therapeutic touch: A holistic tool for nurse practitioners. *Advance for Nurse Practitioners, 10*(5), 69–71.

Carper, B. A. (1975). *Fundamental patterns of knowing in nursing*. Doctoral dissertation, Teachers College, Columbia University. University Microfilms Cat. # 76-7772.

Carper, B. A. (1978). Fundamental patterns of knowing in nursing. *Advances in Nursing Science, 1*(1), 13–23.

Coenen, A., Ryan, P., & Sutton, J. (1997). Mapping nursing interventions from a hospital information system to the Nursing Interventions Classification (NIC). *Nursing Diagnosis, 8*(4), 145–151.

Cumbie, S. A. (2001). The integration of mind-body-soul and the practice of humanistic nursing. *Holistic nursing practice, 15*(3), 56–62.

Daley, B. (1997). Therapeutic touch, nursing practice and contemporary cutaneous wound healing research. *Journal of Advanced Nursing, 25*, 1123–1132.

Dickoff, J., & James, P. (1968). A theory of theories: A position paper. *Nursing Research, 17*, 197–203.

Dingwall, R., & Lewis, P. (Eds.). (1983). *The sociology of the professions*. Cambridge: Macmillan Press.

Donaldson, S. K., & Crowley, D. M. (1978). The discipline of nursing. *Nursing Outlook, 26*, 113–120.

Elasy, T. A., Ellis, S. E., Brown, A., & Pichert, J. W. (2001). A taxonomy for diabetes educational interventions. *Patient Education and Counseling, 43*, 121–127.

Fawcett, J. (1988). Conceptual models and theory development. *Journal of Obstetric, Gynecologic, and Neonatal Nursing, 17*, 400–403.

Feldman, H. R. (1981). A science of nursing—to be or not to be? *Image: Journal of Nursing Scholarship, 13*, 63–66.

Fitzpatrick, J. J. (1987). Use of existing nursing models. *Journal of Gerontological Nursing, 13*(9), 8–9.

Fitzpatrick, J. J. (1988). Theory based on Rogers' conceptual model. *Journal of Gerontological Nursing, 14*(9), 14–16.

Flaskerud, J. H., & Halloran, E. J. (1980). Areas of agreement in nursing theory development. *Advances in Nursing Science, 3*(1), 1–7.

Frederickson, K. (1993). Using a nursing model to manage symptoms: Anxiety and the Roy adaptation model. *Holistic Nursing Practice, 7*(2), 36–43.

Gallop, R., & O'Brien, L. (2003). Re-establishing psychodynamic theory as foundational knowledge for psychiatric/mental health nursing. *Issues in Mental Health Nursing, 24*, 213-227.

Gilje, F. (1992). Being there: An analysis of the concept of presence. In D. A. Gaut (Ed.), *The presence of caring in nursing* (pp. 53-67). New York: NLN Publications (Publication No. 15-2465).

Hardy, M. E. (1978). Perspectives on nursing theory. *Advances in Nursing Science, 1*(1), 27-48.

Hempel, C. G. (1952). *Fundamentals of concept formation in empirical science.* Chicago, IL: University of Chicago Press.

Henry, S. B., Holzemer, W. L., & Miller, T. J. (1997). Comparison of nursing interventions classification and current procedural terminology codes for categorizing nursing activities. *Image: Journal of Nursing Scholarship, 29*, 133-138.

Johnson, D. E. (1959). The nature of a science of nursing. *Nursing Outlook, 7*, 291-294.

Johnson, D. E. (1968). Theory in nursing: Borrowed and unique. *Nursing Research, 17*, 206-209.

Johnson, D. E. (1980). The behavioral system model for nursing. In J. P. Riehl & C. Roy (Eds.), *Conceptual models for nursing practice* (2nd ed.). New York: Appleton-Century-Crofts.

Johnson, M., Maas, M., & Moorhead, S. (Eds.). (2000). *Nursing Outcomes Classification (NOC)* (2nd ed.). St. Louis: Mosby.

Kenny, C. (1994). Nursing intuition: Can it be researched? *British Journal of Nursing, 3*, 1191-1195.

Kim, H. S. (1987). Structuring the nursing knowledge system: A typology of four domains. *Scholarly Inquiry for Nursing Practice, 1*, 111-114.

King, I. M. (1971). *Toward a theory for nursing: General concepts of human behavior.* New York: John Wiley and Sons.

King, I. M. (1981). *A theory for nursing: Systems, concepts, processes.* New York: John Wiley and Sons.

King, L., & Appleton, J. V. (1997). Intuition: A critical review of the research and rhetoric. *Journal of Advanced Nursing, 26*, 194-202.

Kuhn, T. S. (1962). *The structure of scientific revolutions.* Chicago: University of Chicago Press.

Lawson, K. L., & Horneffer, K. J. (2002). Roots and wings: A pilot of a mind-body-spirit program. *Journal of Holistic Nursing, 20*, 250-263.

Levine, M. E. (1966). Adaptation and assessment: A rationale for nursing intervention. *American Journal of Nursing, 66*, 2450-2454.

McCloskey, J. C., & Bulechek, G. M. (Eds.). (2000). *Nursing Interventions Classification (NIC)* (3rd ed.). St. Louis: Mosby-Year Book.

Meehan, T. C. (1998). Therapeutic touch as a nursing intervention. *Journal of Advanced Nursing, 28*, 117-125.

Moorhead, S., & Delaney, C. (1997). Mapping nursing intervention data into the Nursing Interventions Classification (NIC): Process and Rules. *Nursing Diagnosis, 8*(4), 137-144.

Murphy, J. F., & Schmitz, M. (1979). An operationalization of Martha Rogers' theory throughout the nursing process. *International Journal of Nursing Studies, 16*(1), 7-20.

Newman, M. A. (1972). Nursing's theoretical evolution. *Nursing Outlook, 20*, 449-453.

Newman, M. A. (1986). *Health as expanding consciousness.* St. Louis: C. V. Mosby.

Nursing Theories Conference Group. (1980). *Nursing theories : The base for professional nursing practice.* Englewood Cliffs, NJ: Prentice-Hall.

Orem, D. E. (1971). *Nursing: Concepts of practice.* New York: McGraw-Hill.

Orlando, I. (1961). *The dynamic nurse-patient relationship.* New York: G. P. Putnam's Sons.

Paley, J. (1996). Intuition and expertise: Comments on the Benner debate. *Journal of Advanced Nursing, 23*, 665-671.

Parker, M. E. (Ed.). (1991). *Nursing theories in practice.* New York: National League for Nursing.

Parse, R. R. (1981). *Man-living-health: A theory of nursing.* New York: John Wiley & Sons.

Peters, R. M. (1999). The effectiveness of therapeutic touch: A meta-analytic review. *Nursing Science Quarterly, 12*(1), 52-61.

Popper, K. R. (1972). *Conjectures and refutations* (4th ed.). London: Routledge and Kegan Paul.

Rawls, A. C. (1980). Evaluation of the Johnson behavioral model in clinical practice: Report of a test and evaluation of the Johnson theory. *Image: Journal of Nursing Scholarship, 12*(1), 13-16.

Reynolds, P. D. (1971). *A primer in theory construction.* New York: Bobbs-Merrill.

Rodgers, B. L. (1991). Deconstructing the dogma in nursing knowledge and practice. *Image: Journal of Nursing Scholarship, 23,* 177–181.

Rogers, M. E. (1970). *An introduction to the theoretical basis of nursing.* Philadelphia: F. A. Davis.

Rogers, M. E. (1988). Nursing science and art: A prospective. *Nursing Science Quarterly, 1*(3), 99–102.

Roy, C. (1970). Adaptation: A conceptual framework for nursing. *Nursing Outlook, 18,* 42–45.

Roy, C. (1971). Adaptation: A basis for nursing practice. *Nursing Outlook, 19,* 254–257.

Ruffing-Rahal, M. A. (1984). The spiritual dimension of well-being: Implications for the elderly. *Home Healthcare Nurse, 2*(2), 12–13, 16.

Sarvimäki, A., & Stenbock-Hult, B. (1996). Intuition—a problematic form of knowledge in nursing. *Scandinavian Journal of Caring Science, 10,* 234–241.

Schwab, J. (1964a). Structure of the disciplines: Meanings and significances. In G. W. Ford & L. Pugno (Eds.), *The structure of knowledge and the curriculum.* Chicago: Rand McNally.

Schwab, J. (1964b). The structure of the natural sciences. In G. W. Ford & L. Pugno (Eds.), *The Structure of knowledge and the curriculum.* Chicago: Rand McNally.

Sherman, D. W., & Ouelette, S. C. (2001). Patients tell of their images, expectations, and experiences with physicians and nurses on an AIDS-designated unit. *Journal of the Association of Nurses in AIDS Care, 12*(3), 84–94.

Shermis, S. (1962). On becoming an intellectual discipline. *Phi Delta Kappan, 44,* 84–86.

Smith, K. (1997). Let's put the art back into the science of nursing. *Nursing Times, 93*(48), 21.

Steeves, R., Cohen, M. Z., & Wise, C. T. (1994). An analysis of critical incidents describing the essence of oncology nursing. *Oncology Nursing Forum, 21*(Suppl. 8), 19–25.

Thomas, D. V. (2002). Aromatherapy: Mythical, magical, or medicinal? *Holistic Nursing Practice, 16*(5), 8–16.

Thompson, W. Gilman (1908). The over-trained nurse. *New York Medical Journal, 83,* 845–849.

Thoroddsen, A., & Thorsteinssen, H. S. (2002). Nursing diagnosis taxonomy across the Atlantic Ocean: Congruence between nurses' charting and the NANDA taxonomy. *Journal of Advanced Nursing, 32,* 372–381.

Turner, J., Clark, A. J., & Williams, M. (1998). The therapeutic touch on pain and anxiety in burn patients. *Journal of Advanced Nursing, 28,* 10–20.

Uys, L. R. (1980). Towards the development of an operational definition of the concept 'therapeutic use of self'. *International Journal of Nursing Studies, 17,* 175–180.

Visintainer, M. A. (1986). The nature of knowledge and theory in nursing. *Image: Journal of Nursing Scholarship, 18,* 32–38

Watson, J. (1979). *Nursing: The philosophy and science of caring.* Boston: Little, Brown & Co.

Watson, J. (1994). *Applying the art and science of human caring: Introduction.* (Pub. No. 42-2647). New York: National League for Nursing Press.

Watson, J., & Smith, M. C. (2002). Caring science and the science of unitary human beings: A transtheoretical discourse for nursing knowledge development. *Journal of Advanced Nursing, 37,* 452–461.

Watson, M. J. (1988). New dimensions of human caring theory. *Nursing Science Quarterly, 1*(4), 175–181.

Wright, S. M. (1987). The use of therapeutic touch in the management of pain. *Nursing Clinics of North America, 22,* 705–714.

Yamashita, M., Jensen, E., & Tall, F. (1998). Therapeutic touch: Applying Newman's theoretic approach. *Nursing Science Quarterly, 11*(2), 49–50.

CHAPTER 2

Knowledge in Classical Philosophy

KEY IDEAS

cause	induction
cosmologist	intuition
deduction	the one and the many
demonstration	particulars
empiricism	science
essence	skepticism
essentialism	Sophists
forms	syllogism
ideas	universals

The desire to develop nursing knowledge reflects the quest for knowledge that has existed for people throughout history. Aristotle (1947a) astutely pointed out this inherent characteristic of humans in the first line of his work titled *Metaphysics*: "All men [sic] by nature desire to know" (Bk. 1, chap. 1, p. 243). Depending on the historical and social context, knowledge has been desired to gain understanding of the world, to solve relevant problems, or simply for its own sake. Nurses seek knowledge primarily to improve outcomes of care interactions but also to understand their own positions within the broader social and global contexts. Regardless of the focus of knowledge, the ancient Greeks provide a significant historical root for philosophical thought in western civilizations. It is reasonable to start a journey through philosophy and epistemology here for several reasons. The writings and thoughts of the classical philosophers continue to influence much of philosophy and inquiry in contemporary times. One of the more prominent and influential philosophers of this era was Aristotle, a prolific writer who addressed a wide range of topics in his works, for example science, logic, ethics, politics, psychology to name a few. It is a fair indicator of the importance of Aristotle's work in the history of Western thought to note that the current vocabularies of both science and philosophy continue to rely on terminology derived from Aristotle's writings.

A brief overview of the focus of thought during this classical period is necessary to provide the context for a closer look at the work of Aristotle and consequently to provide the foundation for an in-depth look at the evolution of nursing knowledge. In significant contrast to modern views of knowledge and science, the early Greeks saw no distinction between science, knowledge, and philosophy; they sought knowledge primarily for its own inherent value, that is, "knowledge for knowledge's sake." Unlike modern scientists and academics, they were not interested in advancing their particular disciplines or pursuing or expanding existing "theory." But this value does not mean that they sought knowledge primarily through self-reflection or meditation without regard to the world around them. Instead it means they held an intense desire just *to know*.

 ## COSMOLOGY IN ANCIENT GREECE

A common focus for the efforts of the early Greeks to achieve knowledge was the world around them. The early **cosmologists**, known as such because of their interest in understanding the nature of the *cosmos* (the world around them), sought to know what constituted the world—the "stuff"[1] that comprised the world—and how it worked. They recognized that the world around them was constantly changing, as reflected in a statement commonly attributed to Heraclitus, a pre-Socratic Greek philosopher who lived and wrote around the 6th to 5th centuries BCE. (See Box 2-1 for a brief explanation of the abbreviations BCE and CE.) Heraclitus' observation is expressed in a popular paraphrase regarding how it is not possible to step twice into the same river.[2] As presented in the *Fragments*,

> As they step into the same rivers, different and [still] different waters flow upon them. (Heraclitus, Frag. 12, p. 17)

---

[1]The German word *Urstoff* is used in some philosophical writings to capture this idea of "stuff."

[2]Heraclitus' work consists of a variety of original writings and thoughts or ideas generally attributed to him through recollection and anecdote. They have been collected and published as the *Fragments*.

BOX 2-1

BCE AND CE

Many historians and philosophers use the notations BCE and CE, respectively, rather than BC and AD. BCE refers to Before Common Era, and CE refers to the Common Era, or current historical period.

There seemed to be some underlying unity within this constant change and the diversity that the ancients recognized throughout their world. Things change into one element then emerge again in a new form—wood decomposes to dust; from the dust, new life emerges. With so much diversity and change among individual objects in the world, what could account for the unity and harmony that seemed to be present? Similarly nurses often wonder how it is possible to achieve any degree of stability or predictability when people are so different and the world is constantly changing.

Philosophers know this situation of *unity in diversity* as the problem of ***the one and the many***. How do many individual objects manage to function as one, as a whole? Some of the earliest Greek philosophers focused their energies on attempts to identify the substrate that accounted for this unity in an effort to determine a common basis for all that existed in the world. Thales, who lived approximately 636 to 546 BCE, believed that water was the primary "stuff" of the world. Heraclitus (535 to 475 BCE), a cosmologist of this era, viewed the chief substrate as fire,[1] seeing the process of combustion as fundamental to human life as well as to everything else in the world. Anaximenes, who also lived and wrote during this time, argued that the chief substrate was air and viewed air as an intermediary of fire and water. Anaximenes does not hold as prominent a place in history as Thales and Heraclitus, but he deserves to be remembered based on his contributions regarding air as a primary element of the world and his related work on condensation and rarefaction.

The Socratic Era

It is no surprise that the early cosmologists were not successful in uncovering the essence or substrate that all objects had in common and that held the world together, in other words, of solving the problem of the *one* and the *many*. Their lack of success contributed to the development of **skepticism** regarding whether or not it was possible to solve this problem. As a result, philosophers turned their

---

[1]"[The ordered] world, the same for all, no god or man made, but it always was, is, and will be, an ever-living fire, being kindled in measures and being put out in measures." Heraclitus thus provided the basis for the "conflagration theory" of the Stoics (Heraclitus, p. 96; Commentary by Robinson).

focus from nature to an interest in *man*, societies, and customs. This shift to a focus on *man* characterizes the Socratic period; the itinerant teachers during this time became known as the Sophists. The cosmologists had utilized a primarily deductive approach in their quest for knowledge. Working from a foundation provided by general principles and beliefs, the **Sophists** used more of an empirical, inductive model. They aimed to accumulate a wide array of facts, or pieces of information, and then draw on these data to formulate arguments as needed. Unlike the cosmologists, the Sophists did not intend to achieve objective truth; rather, they were interested in practical ends. They traveled throughout Greece teaching a variety of subjects and were particularly known for their teaching of rhetoric.

Following the Persian wars,[1] interest in politics intensified, yet the average person of the time was not prepared to enter or even understand political life. Skills in speaking, argument and persuasion, as would be gained through the study of rhetoric, were invaluable in political pursuits, and recognition of the importance of these abilities provided the Sophists with a willing audience for their teachings. The Sophists, indeed, were skilled orators, able to create an argument to support, or refute, just about anything based on the store of "facts" they accumulated and their powers of rhetoric. This, too, ultimately led to its own form of skepticism, and within a relatively short period of time the label of "sophist" became something to be spurned rather than admired.

This context of skepticism led to the emergence of a new search for knowledge, one premised on certainty and again seeking absolute Truth (see Box 2-2).[2] Socrates was a key figure in this renewed quest. Socrates, whose name commonly is invoked today in regard to a particular form of teaching and inquiry that involves constant questioning, did not produce any of his own ideas or teachings in written form. Thus, what is known about his work comes from his followers, students, and, of course, critics. Plato provides what is one of the best documents regarding Socrates, and Aristotle credits Socrates with two primary contributions: the use of "inductive arguments and universal definitions" (Aristotle, 1958, Book XII, *Metaphysics*).

The Platonic "Forms"

This very brief synopsis of early Greek philosophy shows an initial focus on the external world, a resulting skepticism, a turn toward the person or *man* along with skills for argumentation and rhetoric, and a turn back toward the search for objective truth and understanding of the external world. The problem of the *one and the many*, of unity in diversity, remained and again became the focus of prominent Greek philosophical thought.

---

[1]A series of battles between the Greek States and the Persians occurring approximately 500–449 BCE

[2]Throughout this text, Absolute Truth is written as Truth, while relative truth is presented using all lower case letters.

BOX 2-2

Truth can be referred to generally as Absolute or Relative. Absolute Truth is universally True, without doubt, and not subject to change. Relative truth, in contrast, is truth that is dependent on the context, or "relative" to a specific context or situation. Colloquially, in conversation, Absolute Truth sometimes is referred to as "Big T" Truth, or Truth (with a capital T), with relative truth referred to as "little t" truth. In writing, Absolute Truth might be written as T_A.

Significant in the early work of the cosmologists is not the particular "stuff" these early philosophers identified, but the fact that they attempted to move beyond facts and data to ideas of a universal entity. These early thinkers were not immersed in physical evidence, unlike the scientists of modern[1] times. Like modern people, however, they sought to achieve universal, objective Truth about the world, to be certain about what they knew to the greatest extent possible. An immediate dilemma was confronted, however, in the fact that such infallible knowledge could not be achieved in regard to the physical world. These early philosophers saw empirical reality—that which is available through sensory data, particularly observation or *seeing*—as constantly in flux. Physical objects, which could be observed, were always changing. Consequently the quest for truth and certainty as the basis of knowledge for some of these early philosophers had to be focused on something other than physical reality. This stands in immediate contrast to the usual scientific approach in which science focuses on objects that can be seen or measured. The term **empiricism**, generally equated with *science* in the present day, is derived from the Latin word for experience *(experientia)*, particularly meaning *sensory* experience. Yet the ancient Greeks recognized the limitations associated with a focus on physical reality and sought knowledge on a different level.

Plato's theory of Forms explicitly captures this idea of Truth as existing on a level other than the physical reality of everyday existence. Plato considered knowledge to be concerned with the universal, the ***Ideas*** (as Socrates referred to them) or ***Forms*** (Plato) that constituted the essence of some object. The Ideas or Forms existed in a transcendental realm, a level of existence that surpassed physical reality. Although they could not be seen or touched, Plato saw them as quite real nonetheless; in addition, he argued that they were objective, not based merely on the perception of the person or thinker. Indeed, things that could be seen or touched or measured, as a modern scientist might approach an object, were quite

---

[1]Throughout this book, the term *modern* or *modern science* is used to refer to *modernism* as viewed in philosophy. Chronologically, the Modern period spans from approximately the mid-17th century to the mid-20th century. The characteristics of modernism, sufficient for discussion here, can be gleaned primarily from the discussion of the work of Bacon and the Logical Positivists. See chapters 4 and 6.

fallible because of their constant change. Knowledge could only concern something apart from these objects and could not be obtained by reason alone, that is through the powers of thought and logical argument without any assistance or involvement of the senses.

The Demonstrations of Aristotle

Aristotle built on this foundation provided by Socrates and Plato and provided a philosophy of knowledge that in many respects pervades current ideology. Like many of the philosophers who preceded him in this era, Aristotle did not differentiate among **science**, knowledge, and philosophy. In fact, the terms *philosophy* and *science* were used broadly to address distinct realms of thinking. Through his various works, Aristotle differentiated three branches of science.[1] According to Aristotle, the *speculative* (or theoretical) *sciences* have the goal of creating knowledge; these include "first philosophy" (*metaphysics*), physics, and mathematics, all of which are oriented toward speculating or theorizing. The *practical sciences* are focused on not just knowledge or knowing but also on the ability to *act* in the light of knowledge; these sciences include ethics, politics, and economics. Finally he identified the *productive sciences*, which have a goal of producing something. This realm includes the fine arts, medicine, architecture, rhetoric, and cobbling (shoemaking) as important for the context.

This discussion of the organization of the sciences might be (and has been erroneously) interpreted as comparable to the present day organization of disciplines. Aristotle had no need to develop an argument about disciplines because he saw each of these types of science as clearly related to the others. Unlike contemporary thinkers including nurses who may see at least an organizational or administrative need to separate the sciences, Aristotle emphasized the relationship that existed within all knowledge. Each type of science could be differentiated by means of subject matter, desired end, and basic principles. Yet each is pertinent to the others; principles and subject matter may be shared but are used differently or for different purposes.

Aristotle presents a unique perspective on the current dilemma concerning the organization of knowledge and academic disciplines and sheds some light on recent discussion in nursing about borrowed versus unique knowledge. In this view, knowledge is not the property of any one group or limited to any particular focus; it is shared and developed widely even though the end purposes may differ regarding the reason for creating and using the knowledge. Aristotle also applied the term "science" quite broadly. This is considerably different from current nursing thought that questions whether or not nursing is a science. Such differentiation served no purpose for Aristotle. In fact, the development of *science* as a distinct and especially esteemed form of knowledge is a relatively recent occurrence that is traceable primarily to the early 20th century.

---

[1]See especially Aristotle's writing, *The Topics*.

DIGRESSION FROM PLATO'S THEORY OF FORMS

As noted previously, in regard to the sciences Plato focused on the *Forms* that transcend the realm of actual experience or what might be called the realm of everyday reality. As described by Plato, the forms existed on another level of reality and served as standards or exemplars of which sensible things, the objects we perceive with our senses, were only imperfect copies. Plato argued that knowledge cannot be developed through the senses at all because of the changing and imperfect nature of these sensible objects; instead, the senses could provide only opinion and supposition. This argument provides an example of a lingering dualism in philosophy, the dichotomy concerning *universals* and *particulars*. This dualism recognizes that the world is divided into the separate realities of **particulars** (sensible entities, or objects that can be detected by the senses) and **universals** (abstractions or generalizations that exist apart from the particulars). Immediately a dilemma is created for philosophers: How, then, can knowledge of the universals be obtained? Obviously, according to Plato, knowledge was not created through the senses. As an alternative, Plato suggested that reason, the power of the mind, was suitable for developing this knowledge. But could the mind alone accomplish this? How could such knowledge meet the important criteria of being objective and providing certainty?

Although Aristotle recognized the importance of this problem, he was concerned particularly that Plato's Theory of the Forms significantly separated the objects of everyday reality and the realm of universals. Aristotle scoffed at Plato's notion of *Forms* and sought to unite the world of everyday existence, the *particulars*, with the knowable forms that existed *in* things rather than treating them as separate realms. Creating this union would show how knowledge could be obtained through contact with the objects of everyday experience without the need somehow to surpass the realm in which people live and work on a daily basis. As just a few examples of great interest to nurses, justice, beauty, dignity, and personhood are not objects themselves that need to be examined but are found in objects or particulars present throughout the physical world.

For Aristotle, knowledge was of the universal not the discrete and changing objects around him. But knowledge was acquired through the soul's reception of the forms of *things*, that is, by recognizing the forms that existed in the particulars. The Forms were not to be known through intellectual training, as Plato might have suggested, but could be known through observation and logic (which Aristotle referred to as demonstration). Matter and form were never separated from each other. There could be no pure form without matter, and matter could not exist without form. It seemed inappropriate to discount such experience entirely because people live in a world of empirical existence; they make their way through the world with the use of their senses and are affected by the things they sense. The challenge was to determine how knowledge could be generated through such experience when that experience was changing continuously.

While the world of empirical or sensory experience is important, Aristotle could only give it a relatively low status in relationship to knowledge. According to Aristotle, knowledge focused on the universal; empirical (sensory) experience only provided acquaintance with *particulars*. The gap between universal and particular ultimately calls for some nonempirical element contributed by the mind.

Aristotle provides a radical departure from contemporary (modern) views of science. Typically science today is based on measurement, the senses, facts, the objects around us, what we can observe. Researchers and consumers of science assume that the senses and instruments are accurate, and scientists take great pains to ensure that observations and measurements are standardized and valid. That seen through a microscope and the score obtained on a measure of depression or coping are held to reflect a *real* state of reality. Researchers impose myriad *controls* to keep the mind out of the process; the mind's interjection of any component would be seen as imposing bias on the inquiry, rendering the results subjective rather than objective as desired. However, Aristotle differentiates induction and deduction and shows how the original premise of traditional science and objectivity actually may lead to false conclusions; this is quite the opposite of what is desired and what is presumed accurate.

INDUCTION AND DEDUCTION

Induction can be defined generally as the process of generating a universal conclusion from observation of particulars. When using induction, the investigator examines individual objects and takes measurements of specific, individual instances; using these data, the investigator formulates a more broadly applicable conclusion. In succinct terms, the idea of induction can be regarded as movement from the particular to the general. In contrast, **deduction** involves movement from a general position to a more particular or individualistic one. For example, researchers often develop hypotheses for testing in research through the deduction of the hypotheses from a theory. Following this deductive stage, scientists then usually proceed to the collection of data through induction. Using a process of induction, a nurse might observe that patients who ambulate soon after surgery seem to recover more quickly than those who remain in bed. The nurse might make this observation of a number of individuals and arrive at the more general conclusion that early ambulation is helpful. Working deductively, the nurse would proceed from general principles of physiology along with psychosocial data and support early ambulation as an intervention to promote faster recovery.

In contrast to the typical procedures followed in traditional science, Aristotle argued that induction was inadequate for developing knowledge. A conclusion derived through induction should have the status of universal law because it is applicable on a general level. The conclusion would constitute law, however, which would mean it would be true with certainty if and only if all the particulars had been examined. However, that could never occur because it would be impossible to scrutinize every instance of something. Based on this reasoning, Aristotle argued that induction is not capable of generating scientific proofs.

SYLLOGISMS AND DEMONSTRATIONS

According to Aristotle, the degree of certainty and, therefore, the degree of Truth sought can only be derived through the **syllogism**. The syllogism, a fundamental element of logic, formed the basis for the teaching of traditional formal logic until early in the 20th century when logic assumed a more mathematical orientation. A syllogism consists of three statements: syllogism begins with a premise that is True, applies this premise to an individual or particular instance, then draws a conclusion through logical deduction. Aristotle described the three statements of a syllogism in the following way. First the syllogism starts with the simplest truths, statements so basic it is not possible to demonstrate their truth; these are axioms observable only by the intelligence. The final statement is the more comprehensive truth or general conclusion. The "middle term" sits as a second statement between and connecting these two ends. This middle term is Aristotle's real object of knowledge because it forms the connecting link between the axiomatic truths of the basic premises and the rest of knowledge (Aristotle, 1947b, Book II, pp. 72–109).

An example of a simple syllogism helps to illustrate how Aristotle saw this use of logic contributing to knowledge. First a universal Truth forms the foundation for the syllogism. A statement commonly used for example purposes is the basic premise "all humans are mortal." This statement can be accepted generally as a universal Truth because there has yet to be a human who would not achieve mortality at some point. All available evidence indicates this is a valid, True, statement (at least on a theoretical level not withstanding some future development). Mortality is, in fact, universally True of all humans. Next we might say that Plato was human. Based on what we know about humans, this can be demonstrated by applying ideas of what constitutes "human" to Plato, determining a fit between the characteristics of Plato and those of human, thus determining that Plato was, indeed, human. In other words, Plato displayed the characteristics that comprised the "essence" of human; he possessed the defining criteria for being human. Having established these two parts of the syllogism, we can conclude logically that Plato is mortal. In a written form, the syllogism appears as follows:

All humans are mortal.
Plato is human.
(Therefore,) Plato is mortal.

Philosophers and other practitioners of logic might display the underlying argument in more general terms:

All Ps are Q.
X is P.
X is Q.

Given the Truth of the original premise, it is a necessary fact, meaning that it must be the case, that Plato is mortal. The middle term reveals the "cause" of Plato being mortal: he is mortal because he is human. Where there is an addition to knowledge using this syllogism in this way is in the focus on the middle term, the second line in the syllogism—for Science, according to Aristotle (1947b), is the search for the middle term or **cause** of the thing, because this "cause" is responsible for making the thing what it is:

> We suppose ourselves to possess unqualified scientific knowledge of a thing, as opposed to knowing it in the accidental way in which the sophist knows, when we think that we know the cause on which the fact depends, as the cause of that fact and of no other, and, further, that the fact could not be other than it is. (Book I, chap. 2, p. 11)

Aristotle, therefore, viewed scientific knowledge as *necessary*, which means that the fact simply must be the way it is.

Another example:
Any particular (X) with respiration is organic.
X has respiration.
X is organic.

We know through both observation and deduction that only living (organic) things display a respiratory process. So whenever a particular is identified to have respiration, we know that it can be classified as organic. This property of respiration is a cause of X being organic. Knowing the cause of a thing is knowing its essential nature; uncovering of essence is a major focus of science.

Although many arguments could be constructed in the form of the syllogism, not all syllogisms are equal in strength and value. A syllogism could be constructed as follows, using Aristotle's (1947b, chap. 13, pp. 34–37) example of the apparent "twinkling" of some objects in the night sky:

Things that are near do not twinkle.
The planets are not twinkling.
The planets are near.

This is a **demonstration** of fact because the statements in the syllogism are true for the most part. However, this syllogism does not produce a strong demonstration because it does not properly show the "cause" of the planets' behavior. The planets are not near because they twinkle; twinkling is not the "cause," the proper middle term, for the planets to be near. This syllogism demonstrates the fact but not the *reasoned fact*; its statements and conclusions might be based on sense perception alone.

In this case reversing the major (primary) and middle statements, however, produces a *reasoned fact*.

Things that are near do not twinkle
The planets are near.
The planets do not twinkle.

The superiority of the *reasoned fact* over the mere *fact* is obvious to Aristotle: the middle statement gives the cause of the planets not twinkling, is necessarily true and, therefore, can be posited with certainty.

In addition to preferring the demonstration that shows the *reasoned fact*, Aristotle identified a variety of other criteria for determining the better form of demonstration. In general, the best form of demonstration is one that is "universal and affirmative." Specifically, Aristotle (1947b) directs that preference be given to the demonstration that gives greater knowledge, that fits the universal rather than focusing on a group of particulars, that teaches two things as preferable to that which teaches only one, and that has a "middle term" near to the basic truth, in other words, where there is obviously close dependence between the middle term or *cause* and the basic premise. Aristotle added that the preferable demonstration "touches the real and will not mislead," has a single meaning, "proves the cause," and is independent of other facts. The best form of demonstration also is the simpler and more determinant one, indicating a preference for parsimony and, of course, for Absolute Truth. It is interesting that scientists in a contemporary context also generally seek to generate conclusions that are applicable across a broad variety of situations, that successively reduce diverse and complex ideas into more simple theories, that do so in a parsimonious and comprehensive manner, and that at least approximate certainty or Truth (or have a high probability of being true). In spite of the millennia that have passed since Aristotle's writings, some of his ideas persist in contemporary science.

Aristotle's description of syllogisms and how knowledge can be expanded hinted at the possibility of developing a general classification system with categories and subcategories. This classification approach undoubtedly was influenced to some extent by Aristotle's background and extensive experience in biology. As a taxonomy or other such organizational structure progressively expands, it also provides growing awareness and knowledge of all the elements it contains. Determining the *cause* or **essence** of something, what makes it what *it is*, constitutes the primary focus of science.

Aristotle's idea of *cause*, particularly as it constitutes the *essence* of a thing, appears in another part of his discussion of science regarding "definitions." Aristotle differentiates between nominal and real definitions.[1] While a definition ideally gives the essence or cause of a thing's existence, only a "real" definition fully accomplishes this task. It is not always possible to attain essential or real defini-

---

[1]The distinction between nominal and real definitions is revived in the 1950s by Hempel, a Positivist, and shows great influence on nursing approaches to concept analysis. See chapter 8 in this text.

tions, however, thus descriptive or nominal definitions may be necessary on occasion. Nonetheless, real definitions, according to this ideology, are the only ones that achieve the ideal of knowledge.

One question that invariably arises with Aristotle's discussion of demonstration concerns the origin of the basic premises that form the foundation for syllogisms. These premises, according to Aristotle (1947b), must be

> true, primary, immediate, better known than and prior to the conclusion, which is further related to them as effect to cause. Unless these conditions are satisfied, the basic truths will not be "appropriate" to the conclusion. (Book I, chap. 2, p. 11)

Syllogisms might be created without the premises meeting these conditions, but such a syllogism would not produce scientific knowledge or properly be considered *demonstration* (Book I, chap. 2, pp. 11–12). These premises cannot be demonstrable or they would not be considered primary and basic. The question then arises as to how these are obtained.

Aristotle (1947b) argues that "not all knowledge is demonstrative: on the contrary, knowledge of the immediate premises is independent of demonstration" (Book I, chap. 3, p. 14), as indeed it must be following the argument above. He further points out that these premises are not present "from birth," which would make them innate,

> nor can they come to be in us if we are without knowledge of them to the extent of having no such developed state at all. Therefore, we must possess a capacity of some sort, but not such as to rank higher in accuracy than these developed states. (Aristotle, 1947b, Book II, chap. 19, p. 107)

Instead, Aristotle (1947b) argues that humans can build on an innate faculty present from birth to develop these basic premises through sense-perception. But this is not sense-perception as usually thought in regard to scientific observation. Rather sense-perception contributes an impression on the mind or a memory, the "remaining of the percept" that persists when the actual perception ends. From this memory comes experience based on repeated memory, or the fixation of a universal:

> From the universal now stabilized in its entirety within the soul, the one beside the many which is a single identity within them all—originate the skill of the craftsman and the knowledge of the man of science, skill in the sphere of coming to be and science in the sphere of being. (Book II, chap. 19, pp. 107-108)

These basic premises arise through a process of induction, through sense-perception of individuals (particulars) on a repeated basis such that "the earliest universal is present in the soul: for though the act of sense-perception is of the particular, its content is universal..." (Book II, chap. 19, p. 108). Through repeated confrontation with particulars, "indivisible concepts, the true universals, are established..." (Book II, chap. 19, p. 108–109). This process of induction is not a systematic process of data gathering as a modern day scientist might pursue. Instead Aristotle compares this form of induction to **intuition**, where the universal is immediately present to the thinker. It is "intuition that apprehends the primary premises." Intuition is the only form of knowledge that is as true, perhaps more true than the "scientific knowledge" obtained through demonstration. Therefore, the primary premises are an appropriate basis for the demonstrations that produce scientific knowledge. Intuition, therefore, forms the basis or "originative source" (Book II, chap. 19, p. 109) for scientific knowledge.

In a later part of his work, Aristotle (1947b) describes specifically what he considers to be the right method of investigation. This method begins with observation of a group of "identical individuals"—in other words, a set of particulars that have a specific feature in common. Through examination and application of demonstration to this set, the inquirer determines what they have in common, and what is the "cause" or essence of the common characteristic. Inquiry proceeds to examination of another set of particulars that is related but not identical with the set examined first. In other words, once a particular feature or characteristic is grasped or known, the investigator expands the scope of inquiry to examine that feature in other similar sets. The inquiry shall "persevere until we reach a single formula, since this will be the definition of the thing" (Book II, chap. 13. p. 99). This process resembles the biological work of Aristotle, cataloging an extensive array of items and developing a taxonomic system for categorization. Using a combination of inductive and deductive strategies, Aristotle's ideas reveal a systematic approach to gain objective knowledge, the absolute Truth about the world. Operating from basic premises secured through a complex process of sense perception, memory, and experience of the universal, knowledge can be expanded to progressively demonstrate the essences of aspects of the world and achieve the level of certainty appropriate to distinguish knowledge from opinion.

Influence of Aristotle

The specific details of Aristotle's ideas and methods for gaining knowledge are intriguing, impressive, and quite advanced compared to what many readers might expect for his time. Although he lived and worked nearly 2500 years ago, Aristotle's contributions to philosophy and his influence have endured. It is also important to point out as well that he and his contemporaries confronted some of the same questions that currently perplex modern nurses. The problem of unity in diversity, of the one and the many, is not far removed from nurses' own values and beliefs in a dynamic and changing nature of the world and of people and the difficulties inherent in trying to capture events and meaning in a changing context. Nurses also have struggled with ways to study and gain knowledge of things that are not amenable to traditional empirical study yet that hold important places in the intellectual history of nursing. Some examples of these nonempirical entities are spirituality, energy, resilience, hardiness, "becoming," and "presence"; these are just a few of the abstract concepts important in nursing practice. Perhaps even "health" could be added to the list. Aristotle's approach to knowledge is focused on nonempirical entities as well, the universals, although the methodology he proposed is intended to show how such nonempirical elements might be accessed or known through a combination of observation and logical argument (demonstration).

Intuition often is used to explain some of nurses' knowledge and skill, particularly when empirical cues for actions are not obvious. Aristotle provides an interesting perspective on intuition that may enlighten discussion of its role in nursing knowledge. According to Aristotle, this human capacity is used to grasp the basic premises that provide the foundation for demonstrations. Although the grasp of these basic premises is derived from sense-perception, the credibility of these premises goes beyond the acts of mere seeing or perceiving. In describing this process of arriving at the basic principles, Aristotle sheds some light on the process of intuition and certainly its value in developing knowledge; this raises interesting questions as well about the combination of inductive and deductive strategies in the quest for knowledge.

For Aristotle, the claims to knowledge that resulted from these processes had to be irrefutable, certain, and necessary. This end product would meet the criteria for objective, Absolute Truth. Aristotle referred to this product as "science," creating a foundation for viewing science as systematic, objective, and Truth-seeking. He did not see this as different from knowledge in general, however, and in fact substituted the term "science" for "knowledge" on occasion. The roots of Western philosophy, as evidenced in the classical period of Greece, have a strong thread addressing knowledge using terms such as Truth, necessity, and certainty. However, it is worth noting that "science" is not always considered as a distinct and specific subset of knowledge with unique goals and criteria.

Aristotle's "science" and Truth, however, are focused on "essences." For Aristotle, an essence is whatever makes something what it is. Essence is the "cause" of the thing, that which makes the particular thing what it is and not something else. The search for knowledge (science) in this approach is focused on uncovering the "essence" of the things examined, that is, what makes a particular an example of animal, beauty, justice, organic. When the "essence" is found and has been determined necessarily connected to the object, it can be said that the "cause" of the thing has been found, according to Aristotle. This is Aristotle's "science." This idea of **essentialism** has persisted through modern times in various forms in the idea that an essence can be discovered and reflects a single, objective reality or Truth about an object or experience. Various philosophers subsequently have explored the virtues, and problems associated with ideas such as "essence" and "necessity."[1]

It is questionable, indeed unlikely, that the procedures described by Aristotle actually could result in the objective knowledge sought by this prominent philoso-

---

[1]See, for example, Kripke S. A. (1980). *Naming and necessity*. Oxford: Basil Blackwell, and Plantinga, A. (1965). *The ontological argument*. New York: Doubleday.

pher. Could the basic premises really be grasped with complete accuracy, free from possible error or bias? Aristotle undoubtedly believed that it was possible to achieve such Truth about the world and put forth his idea of the proper form of investigation to reach this goal. His method, a unique blend of inductive and deductive and of the universal and the particular, is an attempt to gain knowledge of the world in which he and his contemporaries lived.

Through his writings Aristotle provided the history of Western intellectual thinking with a plethora of terms and ideas, many of which continue to influence epistemology and science in much of the world. For nurses, it is particularly interesting to note the advancement of his times, for example, the effort to construct taxonomies, to understand the planets and moons, and to construct knowledge of the world around them some 5 or 6 centuries ago, just as contemporary societies struggle to do. There is great similarity in the ideas of change and the struggle to unite the realms of everyday particulars with a realm in which objective, universal knowledge might exist. Similarly there is a search for methods to achieve the intellectual goals of the era. While the problems addressed might be radically different, the desire to know and the questions about what constitutes knowledge persist.

 ## CONCLUSION

Nurse scholars should be able to appreciate the similarities between some of the challenges confronted by Aristotle and those in nursing. Much of nursing science has developed during a time of ideology that distinguishes between science and other forms of knowledge, induction and deduction, empiricism and intuition, and that has contributed to other similar dichotomies in discussions of inquiry. While many of these distinctions are legitimate, Aristotle provides considerable incentive for considering that a combination of perception and logical reasoning can contribute to the growth of knowledge. The human mind possesses many faculties with which to know the world. Aristotle encourages thinking about how, through a combination of powers and abilities, it is possible to know much about the surrounding world despite its dynamic and changing nature.

 ## FOR DISCUSSION

1. How does the problem of "the one and the many" relate to nursing?
2. Describe an *idea* or universal in nursing and how it might be discovered through examination of everyday experience.
3. Discuss strengths and weaknesses of sensory data in the development of knowledge.
4. Construct a syllogism to demonstrate a Truth relevant to nursing.

REFERENCES

Aristotle. (1947a). Metaphysics (Book I) (W. D. Ross, Trans.). In R. McKeon (Ed.), *Introduction to Aristotle* (pp. 238–243). New York: Random House.

Aristotle. (1947b). Analytica Posteriora (Books I & II) (G. R. G. Mure, Trans.). In R. McKeon (Ed.), *Introduction to Aristotle* (pp. 9–109). New York: Random House.

Aristotle. (1958). *Metaphysics: A revised text with introduction and commentary by W. D. Ross* (W. D. Ross, Trans.). Oxford: Clarendon Press.

Heraclitus. (1987). *Fragments*. (T. M. Robinson, Trans.). Toronto: University of Toronto Press. (Original work 5th/6th Century BCE)

CHAPTER 3

Knowledge from Within: The Rationalism of Descartes

KEY IDEAS

body	mind
dualism	private and public worlds
idea	rationalism
innate ideas	reason

One major contribution to Western epistemology came with the work of the French philosopher, Rene Descartes. Although Descartes lived and wrote during the 17th century, it is important to recognize that the period between the 4th century BCE, which was the time of Classical philosophy and the work of Aristotle, and 17th century Europe certainly was not a time of inactivity. Thinkers of this extended period continued to explore the major questions posed in earlier Greek philosophy and to experience the influence of the classics. The intervening time saw the hedonistic ethics of Epicurus, the nominalism of William of Ockham,[1] and ultimately the great intellectual movement of the Renaissance

---

[1]Epicurus supported the idea of atoms as the basic components of physical matter, an idea derived from the pre-Socratic philosopher Democritus. This atomism contributed to a decidedly empirical focus for knowledge. Epicurus also is associated with a hedonistic approach to ethics, arguing that behavior occurs generally in the pursuit of pleasure. Ockham's nominalism asserts, in general, a rejection of metaphysical universals and a reduction of metaphysical categories to the most parsimonious possible. Ockham did not support the existence of universals as individual entities; universal only meant applicable to many instances.

during the 14th and 15th centuries CE, beginning in Italy and spreading westward across Europe.

Prior to Descartes a period of emerging religious rule was controversial in the stark contrast with the great advances of science. For example during the time of William of Ockham in the 14th century, empirical research concomitant with developments in psychology combined to create an interest in and focus on reason in the field of epistemology; this also generated a conflicting recognition that nature dealt primarily with particulars (empirical objects). Science was thought to be focused on propositions and general concepts that exist only in the mind rather than with things themselves or physical objects. This tension between the mind and external reality led ultimately to the need for workable theories of knowledge to address adequately the ways in which sensory data obtained through interaction with particulars would contribute to the development of concepts of these objective realities.

OVERVIEW OF DESCARTES' PHILOSOPHY

Historical Influences

Although there is little direct link between the works of Ockham and Descartes, the developments that preceded the work of Descartes clearly had a significant effect on shaping his ideas and establishing the context for his writing. Descartes worked against the backdrop formed by religion, science, and a rising attention to theories of knowledge. He was schooled heavily in the classics yet subsequently rejected most of those teachings. He lived and worked during the time of great religious influence yet also during the era of Galileo. The facts that no one had seen God through a telescope and that the Copernican system of astronomy generated tremendous disputes about religion and science threatened a new skepticism that would undermine both religion and science (see Box 3-1). Descartes saw his challenge in devising the method that would provide appropriate grounds for the existence of knowledge, in other words, a method that would make it possible to generate conclusions that would count as "knowledge."

Development of Method

Descartes is well known for his work in the area of mathematics and is credited with developing a system of coordinate geometry. In regard to philosophy, he is credited with leaving the enduring legacy of the "Cartesian dualism," or the "mind–body **dualism**." However, this legacy often is misunderstood and the frequent reference to Descartes regarding only this "dualism" presents a superficial portrayal of his philosophical work.

BOX 3-1

IMPACT OF COPERNICAN ASTRONOMY

In simple terms, Copernican astronomy presents the planets as revolving around the sun. Previously the dominant belief (the Ptolemaic system) had been that the earth was the center of the universe and the sun and other elements revolved around the earth. This change in relationship of the planets and the sun raised questions about the relationship between heaven and Earth; this view was contrary to the teachings of Scripture and regarded widely at the time as patently false and lacking any scientific proof. Galileo, a talented mathematician, supported the Copernican system and invented his version of the telescope in 1609 to further study astronomy. He was subsequently tried and condemned by the Roman Catholic Church and sent into exile primarily for failure to obey the previous orders of the church that he was not to teach his astronomic views. Pope John Paul II recanted the previous action against Galileo in 1992 although debate about the significance of this entire sequence of events still lingers.

Descartes' fundamental desire to provide the method for obtaining knowledge was the major driving force of his work. This method is described succinctly in his work *Discourse on Method* (1637/1976b). Here Descartes provides the following rules for the development of knowledge:

> The first of these was to accept nothing as true which I did not clearly recognize to be so; that is to say, carefully to avoid precipitation and prejudice in judgments, and to accept in them nothing more than what was presented to my mind so clearly and distinctly that I could have no occasion to doubt it.
>
> The second was to divide up each of the difficulties which I examined into as many parts as possible, and as seemed requisite in order that it might be resolved in the best manner possible.
>
> The third was to carry on my reflections in due order, commencing with objects that were the most simple and easy to understand, in order to rise little by little, or by degrees, to knowledge of the most complex, assuming an order, even if a fictitious one, among those which do not follow a natural sequence relatively to one another.
>
> The last was in all cases to make enumerations so complete and reviews so general that I should be certain of having omitted nothing. (Descartes, 1637/1976b, *Discourse on Method,* part II, p. 118)

Keeling (1934) points out that these rules rely on three distinct mental operations: intuition, deduction, and enumeration. As presented by Aristotle, intuition is the immediate apprehension of the simplest nature of an object. For Descartes deduction was not a syllogistic demonstration but a means of deducing relationships among the simple natures. Enumeration provides a means to organize aspects of deduction to avoid error.

While Descartes' method had its proponents, critics such as the famed mathematician Pierre de Fermat dismissed it.[1] Taken by themselves, the rules are so general and essential terminology so vague that they provide little guidance in the quest for knowledge. Possibly Descartes would have admitted that his "rules" are abstract prescriptions with little substantive content. He emphasized repeatedly that the *application* of the mind to specific problems made it possible to have knowledge, to see something "clearly and distinctly." This meaning of "clear and distinct" (Descartes,1637/1976b, *Discourse on Method*, pp. 118, 128) perception is one of the central issues in the interpretation of the method and is certainly a central concern for Descartes. It is this idea of "clear and distinct" that provides the impetus for his more elaborate work on the method, the well-known *Meditations on First Philosophy* (Descartes, 1641/1976c).

Knowledge exists when there are "clear and distinct ideas" according to Descartes. To determine what clear and distinct ideas exist, Descartes employs his method of doubt, setting aside anything that can be supposed false until the mind arrives at something that cannot be supposed false. In other words, ideas are subjected to doubt and the attempt to view them as false until it is no longer possible for the idea to be false. There, at last, the mind arrives at the degree of truth and certainty that enables the idea to be considered knowledge.

This process of doubting might seem to resemble a form of skepticism. However, Descartes clearly is not a skeptic in that he has a definite idea that knowledge is possible, what it is, and how to acquire it. To begin this process, Descartes identifies a beginning point with one proposition that cannot be doubted, that he cannot be wrong in maintaining: *Ego sum, ego existo*. This proposition translates to *I am, I exist*. In Part IV of the *Discourse on Method* (1637/1976b) he elaborates on this proposition by stating *cogito ergo sum, I think, therefore I am* (p. 127). For Descartes, the fact that he is thinking necessarily means that he exists, otherwise he could not be aware of his thought processes. In other words, how could Descartes possibly be aware of his own thinking if he did not exist, if his idea of himself were false or illusion?

Descartes' emphasis on his own conscious processes, which is referred to as the *cogito*, is an important foundation for his thesis on knowledge and leads him to two significant conclusions. First, the "I" in his statement is a substance whose whole essence is to *think* (*Discourse on Method*, 1637/1976b, p. 128). What makes it possible for him to be certain of his own existence is the fact that he has thought processes. These thought processes thus make him the *I* that he knows. Second,

---

[1]Fermat, a noted French mathematician, is considered to be the founder of modern number theory and a major developer of probability theory. The equation known as Fermat's Last Theorem (that $x^N + y^N = z^N$, where x, y, z, and N are integers other than zero and has no solutions for N greater than 2) occupied mathematicians for several hundred years in their attempts to construct proofs for this theorem.

this thinking substance is "really distinct" from any physical body he has. Descartes can be certain of his existence as a thinking thing while still in doubt that he has a body. Based on this realization, he and his body—if he has one—must be really distinct from one another.

The "real distinction" between the mind and the body is one of the central doctrines of the meditations. Over time real distinction has become a lasting legacy of Descartes' work and one that pervades much of nursing and related medical activity. Descartes, in fact, is widely remembered for this "Cartesian dualism" created by the juxtaposition of the mind and the body. This often is regarded a bit superficially as the "separation" of the **mind** and **body**. Yet Descartes has not addressed any separation as yet, only that the mind and body are different.

Distinction of Body and Mind

Still, Descartes' distinctions give rise to some perplexing questions regarding the relationship of the mind and the body. Over time it is clear that scientists pursued the mind and body as separate, sometimes only questionably related; this contributed to rather excessive separations among physiological and behavioral approaches to human beings. This distinction is particularly evident in health care where biological theories often have been at great odds with behavioral theories of health and illness; nurses are quite familiar with the lingering "nature vs. nurture" ideas about human development.

This degree of separation, however, is not wholly consistent with Descartes' views. In *Passions of the Soul*, (1649/1989), Descartes acknowledges that there must be a fusion of mind and body to make a human being. The mind and the body both could exist without the other and can act independently of each other. A human being, however, involves the union of both. To explain precisely how this union is derived, Descartes points to the pineal gland as the source of fusion between the mind and the body (*Passions of the Soul,* 1649/1989, part 1). According to Descartes, the soul (mind) directly moves the pineal gland, thus directly affecting the "animal spirits" (which are the source of mechanical changes in the body). Descartes' focus on the role of the pineal gland in this process seems coincidental; his argument for the union of mind and body through some mechanism is the crucial observation here. It is perhaps of historical interest, however, to note that Descartes selected the pineal gland because of its uniqueness in the brain; there is only one pineal gland though the human has two of other body parts including hands, eyes, and ears. The presence of only one such structure made it seem a logical site for performing the union of two disparate components, the body and mind. Descartes also believed, albeit falsely, that other animals did not have such a gland. Therefore, it seemed that this must be the source of the fusion of mind and body. Nonetheless, Descartes did go to a great extent to reinforce his argument regarding the differences between the mind and the body,

> that the whole nature of the mind consists in thinking, while the whole nature of the body consists in being an extended thing, and that there is nothing at all common to thought and extension... The mind can act independently of the brain... (*Objections and Replies*, 1967, p. 212)

This notion of the soul *in* the body creates an image of the invisible soul driving the body as a ghost might direct a machine. Descartes hoped to avoid such an impression, however, and pointed out that the body can do many things on its own; yet the soul feels pain, touch, heat, and other sensations that clearly are in the body. It is not the mere physical separation of the mind and the body that Descartes proposes but also the uniqueness of each aspect:

> First, I hold that there are in us certain primitive notions, which are like the models on whose pattern we form all other knowledge...we have, specifically for body, only the notion of extension, from which are derived the notions of figure and motion. And for the soul alone, we have only the notion of thought, in which are included the conceptions of the understanding and the inclinations of the will. Finally, for soul and body together, we have only the notion of their union, from which are derived our notions of the power which the soul has to move the body, and the body to act on the soul, to cause feelings and passions. (Descartes, 1976a, *Correspondence with Princess Elizabeth*, p. 374)

Descartes notes that there are only two essential attributes in the world; that is, the two characteristics of thought and extension that necessarily apply to anything that exists. Thought, of course, is the essential property of thinking things (the mind or soul). In contrast, physical things have the property that they can be *extended*, which means they can occupy space. This distinction of these two types of characteristics has significant implications for the development of western science. Surely if mind and body had unique characteristics, there would be distinct ways to study them. Before continuing that discussion, however, it is necessary first to continue with an explanation of whether or not the body really exists.

Descartes uses this argument about the uniqueness of the mind and the body to form the foundation for the remainder of his thesis to show with certainty that a physical world exists. In other words given only his consciousness, his power of cognition or thought, how can he be certain that there is a world that exists outside his mind? Descartes attempts to accomplish this objective by proving the existence of God. The existence of other things, an external world, is based on Descartes idea of "God" as a perfect and infinite being without error or defect. The existence of images and sensations of an external reality does not show without doubt that the external reality actually exists. Humans, however, have a strong natural tendency to believe that the external world exists. According to Descartes, if there were not such a reality then it would mean that God had created creatures that were continually misled. This would cause God to appear as a deceiver, which is certainly not accurate given God's perfection, according to Descartes. Therefore, following this line of argument, Descartes concludes without doubt that the external world exists.

Knowledge of the External World

Obviously people do make mistakes; for example, they misjudge things, see things that are not real, or see things as different from what they really are. Descartes accounts for such errors as the result of human free will not as related to any deception by God. According to Descartes, God guides the person toward what is true and what is good. The person must be willing to be guided appropriately; however, error still may be the result based on individual free will. Errors, therefore, are not related to any flaws on the part of God but are the result of free will on the part of humans.

Descartes believes he has proven both that an external world exists and that it is possible to have knowledge of that exterior reality based on the existence of God and the capabilities bestowed upon humans. A final significant doctrine of Descartes' work concerns precisely how such knowledge is obtained. Descartes' views are in complete opposition to traditional ideas of knowledge in the context of modern science where knowledge of physical reality is obtained through empirical, or sensory, data. For Descartes, it is not possible to have knowledge of the physical world in this way. Descartes (1641/1976c) presents an elaborate scenario concerning the melting of wax to demonstrate his point about the impossibility of knowledge based on empirical or sensory data (*Meditations II*, pp. 175–178). He asks the reader to consider a piece of wax that is taken freshly from a hive and still with the sweetness of honey and the odor of the flowers. Descartes describes this scenario: as Descartes moves closer to the fire he is sitting near, the wax loses its smell, taste, form—all the physical attributes it seemed to possess on first inspection. This melting of the wax demonstrates the changeable nature of the physical world. Clearly Descartes could not *know* the wax by reference to its physical character alone; that has been altered radically. Yet the wax has not disappeared; Descartes still can view an object in his hand even though the once firm and easily contained wax is now in a liquid, flexible form. The senses do not provide knowledge of the wax. It is the "mind alone which perceives [the wax]" (Descartes, 1641/1976c, *Meditations II*, p. 176); this perception "is neither an act of vision, nor of touch, nor of imagination, ... but only an intuition of the mind..." (p. 177). Building on this description, Descartes calls for the rejection of sensory data just as he suggested the rejection of all of his former opinions as a means to free his mind for discovery of that which is true.

In contrast to sensory data, Descartes (1641/1976c) argues that knowledge is based on **"innate ideas."** These ideas are "pure," devoid of sensory material and created by God along with the soul or mind. These "innate ideas" are not mere reproductions of sensory experience; they exist on a level totally removed from sense data. Descartes provides one example of an innate *idea* by describing how sitting in proximity to a fire will produce the sensation and subsequently the idea of heat in an individual even if the individual has no prior knowledge of heat. The resulting idea of heat also will occur regardless of the individual's will because the idea of heat will be conjured whether or not the individual wills for that to happen (*Meditations II*, p. 182). Similarly pain may be an example of an "innate idea" because it can be invoked in many instances without the individual having any prior experience of pain.

Implications

This brief overview of Descartes' philosophy points to some of the critical aspects of his work that have had a lasting legacy in philosophy and epistemology. One unique feature obviously is the defining characteristic of **Rationalism**. Cartesian rationalism concerns the overriding focus of **reason** as the source of knowledge. In an extreme form, a Rationalist view holds that all that is or can be known is known through a process of mental reasoning. Rationalism thus also holds that there are truths that can be known without any prior experience of these truths. Such truths are referred to as *a priori* truths based on the fact that they are known *prior* to any experience of them.

The recognition of these truths is dependent to some extent on the ideas that are innate in the mind. In fact, one of Descartes greatest contributions to discussions of knowledge was his notion of "**idea**." Descartes introduced "ideas" as something that exist as the focus of thought. This emphasis on ideas as the essence of thought is derived to some extent from his argument concerning distinctions between the mind and the body or between the thinking substance and the extended, physical substance of the body. An extension of this dualism is the distinction between "**private**" and "**public**" **worlds**. The mind with its content of ideas and its powers of thought is distinctly "private," known only to the individual thinker. In contrast, the body is accessible to the public because it is extended (takes up space); others can observe or feel this physical entity and coexist with it with their own bodies.

For purposes of developing knowledge, the accessibility of the body due to its physical presence seems to make it far more amenable to inquiry. A scientist can observe, measure, and use similar sensory mechanisms to collect information about the body that is likely to be replicable and of good quality. The mind, however, is uniquely private and, therefore, not amenable to such empirical data collection. The result of this distinction has been a seemingly intractable barrier to the study of the mind and the creation of additional dualisms related to differences between the physical and mental realms of existence.

Criticisms and Objections

This distinction between body and mind also was the focus of much criticism and commentary that Descartes received following the publication of the *Meditations*. Pierre Gassendi, a prominent priest and mathematician of the time, presented a particularly lengthy set of objections (known as the Fifth objections) that should be of interest to modern scientists particularly for their materialistic foundation. Gassendi (1641/1967), for example, raised questions concerning both the ambiguous use of the terms "soul" and "mind" as well as about Descartes' argument that the essence of the mind is to think. In his response to Gassendi, Descartes reiterated his notion of the mind as a thinking thing while the "whole nature of the body consists in being an extended thing, and that there is nothing at all common to thought and extension" (Descartes, 1967, *Objections and Replies*, p. 212). Descartes proceeded to explain how he saw the mind as distinct from the brain and able to "act independently of the brain; for certainly the brain can be of no use in pure thought: its only use is for imaging and perceiving" (Descartes, *Objections and Replies*, p. 281–282). Gassendi further criticized, as did many of Descartes objectors, the notion of "clear and distinct ideas," the union of the mind and the body, and Descartes' view of knowledge. The latter, which ties the notion of Truth to clear and distinct ideas ("that all things which I perceive very clearly and very distinctly are true"), evoked the following response from Gasssendi (1641/1967):

> But though amid the obscurity that surrounds us, there may very well be no bet-
> ter Rule obtainable, yet when we see that many minds of the first rank, which
> seem to have perceived many things so clearly and distinctly, have judged that
> the truth of things is hidden either in God or in a well, may it not be open to
> us to suspect that the Rule is perhaps fallacious? (p. 151)

Gassendi cautioned Descartes that he "ought not so much to take pains to substantiate this Rule [of clear and distinct ideas], following which we so readily mistake the false for the true, as to propound a method which will direct us and show us when we are in error and when not, so often as we think that we clearly and distinctly perceive anything" (p. 152).

Gassendi points out a chief flaw in Descartes' argument: Descartes does not demonstrate how we can ever be certain that any idea is "clear and distinct" and there is no guarantee that the idea is necessarily true even if that demonstration were done. Descartes also places tremendous reliance on his notion of God who, as Descartes describes, is not a deceiver. It is primarily this view of the nature of God that makes the discernment of "clear and distinct" ideas possible.

Noted philosopher Richard Rorty (1979) also criticized the distinction ("separation") of mind from body proposed by Descartes in regard to the notion of "extended substance" (p. 62). Rorty pointed out a compelling rebuttal to Descartes' claims using Descartes' own example of pain "in" an amputated limb (a situation nurses immediately recognize as phantom limb pain). Descartes argued that such pain (or such an idea of pain) clearly was not specifically grounded because if it were embodied, it would be pain *in* the limb although the limb no longer exists. Rorty pointed out the awkwardness of considering "a thought or a pain as a *thing* (a particular distinct from a person, rather than a state of a person) which was not locatable unless we already had the notion of a nonextended substance of which it might be a portion" (p. 63). Nonetheless, "contemporary philosophy of mind finds itself talking about *pains* and *beliefs* rather than *people having* pains or beliefs" (p. 63).

Other aspects of Descartes' philosophy equally are open to criticism. Numerous philosophers have criticized Descartes' argument that it is not possible to distinguish the state of being awake from the state of dreaming without appeal to the powers of God (Haldane & Ross, 1967). Combined with other weaknesses in his writings, Descartes certainly failed to accomplish his intended purpose with the *Meditations*, which was "to put forth an argument for the existence and nature of God and the soul on philosophical, rather than theological grounds" (Descartes, 1641/1976c, *Meditations*, p. 154).

Contributions to Modern Science

Descartes did, nonetheless, make a significant contribution to epistemology and to subsequent developments that became modern science. His emphasis on thought serves as a cornerstone for a philosophical position known as Rationalism. In a colloquial context, being "rational" means being logical or reasonable in action or thought. In philosophy, the tradition of Rationalism advocates that the power of Reason, of the mind, is the source of knowledge. For Descartes, the truths derived through reason are not constructed solely by the powers of the mind; instead they likely would be deduced from the ideas that are innate. As noted previously, Descartes' notion of ideas has been the foundation for much philosophical discussion about the mind and thought throughout modern times. Much of scientific contemporary views are derived from debate about whether or not knowledge is even partly created by the mind and the extent to which sensory data has value in the creation of knowledge.

Descartes' dualism of mind and body is significant for nurses and others who study human beings; this longstanding legacy continues to influence both what about human beings can be studied and understood as well as the methods appropriate for such study. Descartes' presentation of a way in which knowledge might be obtained without the observation and measurement required of typical empirical approaches is also of interest to nurses. This process of doubt and reason begins with the rejection of prior beliefs; this frees the mind of the confusion and dogma that cloak it from obtaining knowledge.

CONCLUSION

While many philosophers and especially scientists may be primarily concerned with what is True, it is worth noting that Descartes' emphasis was on the method for developing knowledge. Descartes presented a systematic and rigorous method for the development of knowledge. These criteria continue to be important in discussions about thought and knowledge. Phenomena or characteristics of interest to nurses, such as dignity, quality, support, and justice, are studied using traditional scientific approaches only by providing strict operational definitions of the phenomena and means to measure them. However, Descartes places value on the powers of the mind and rational thought to gain knowledge, not on the senses and measurement. In view of the importance of such phenomena in nursing, other approaches to inquiry are worth considering. The possibility that the powers of the mind, once freed from authority and tradition, could equal or exceed those of scientific instruments is an intriguing project for nursing research.

FOR DISCUSSION

1. Construct an argument to support the statement that you are awake and exist.
2. Discuss examples of the distinction between mind and body in nursing practice.
3. Discuss ways in which the distinction of mind and body has influenced nursing research.
4. Identify ways in which this distinction might be avoided in nursing practice and research.
5. Discuss strengths and weaknesses of reason as a means to develop knowledge. Compare these identified characteristics to thoughts about sensory data.

REFERENCES

Descartes, R. (1967). Objections and replies. *The philosophical works of Descartes*, Vol. 2. (E. S. Haldane & G. R. T. Ross, Trans.). Cambridge: University of Cambridge Press.

Descartes, R. (1976a). Correspondence with Princess Elisabeth. In M. D. Wilson (Ed.), *The essential Descartes* (pp. 373–380). New York: Penguin Books. (Original work published 1643).

Descartes, R. (1976b). Discourse on the method of rightly conducting one's reason and seeking truth in the sciences. In M. D. Wilson (Ed.), *The essential Descartes* (pp. 106–153). New York: Penguin Books. (Original work published 1637).

Descartes, R. (1976c). Meditations on first philosophy. In M. D. Wilson (Ed.), *The essential Descartes* (pp. 154–223). New York: Penguin Books. (Original work published 1641).

Descartes, R. (1989). *Passions of the Soul.* (S. Voss, Trans.). Indianapolis, IN: Hackett. (Original work published 1649).

Gassendi, P. (1967). The fifth set of objections: Letter from P. Gassendi to M. Descartes. In E. S. Haldane & G. R. T. Ross (Trans.), *The philosophical works of Descartes*, Vol. 2. (pp. 135–203) Cambridge: University of Cambridge Press. (Original work published 1641).

Haldane, E. S., & Ross, G. R. T. (1967). *The philosophical works of Descartes*, Vols 1 & 2. Cambridge: University of Cambridge Press.

Keeling, S. V. (1934). *Descartes.* London: Benn.

Rorty, R. (1979). *Philosophy and the mirror of nature.* Princeton, NJ: Princeton University Press.

CHAPTER 4

The Road to Modern Science: British Empiricism

KEY IDEAS

a priori	physical realism
complex idea	probability
concept	proof
empiricism	reflection
experience	sensation
idea	simple idea
impression	skepticism
knowledge	*tabula rasa*

The empiricists of 17th and 18th century Britain provide much of the foundation for how science is viewed in modern times. The philosophers of this group, who typically are referred to as the British Empiricists, are George Berkeley, John Locke, and David Hume (actually of Scottish origin). Defined very broadly, **empiricism** is a philosophy that holds that all knowledge stems from experience. The word *empiricism* is a variation of the Latin term *empeiria*, which is derived from the Greek word for *experience*. In common language, **experience** often is thought of as a personal encounter with a situation; this includes the emotional, subjective, and personal meanings that are attached to the situation and that help to comprise the total experience. *Experience* has a much more specialized meaning for empiricists, however, who view experience specifically in regard to *sensory data*, or information gathered through the senses. The rise of empiricism represents a strong contrast to earlier philosophies, particularly those of Descartes and the scholars of the classical period. Plato and others, for example, argued that sensory data could not provide us with any knowledge but that knowledge transcended the realm of the physical world. In an effort to show how sensory data could contribute to knowledge, Aristotle argued for the combination of induction with the systematic process of demonstration. This process involved a cognitive component as a way of uniting the physical and nonphysical worlds in an effort to gain knowledge. However, Aristotle very clearly argued that while the senses provide useful data, they could not be relied upon for knowledge nor are a source of knowledge. Descartes also was strong in his position that the senses were not a source of knowledge; he argued that knowledge came from the mind alone in part from ideas innate to every human being. The Empiricists, however, argued against these positions and supported the idea that sensory experience is the source of all knowledge (Box 4-1).

The time of the British Empiricists was one of global expansion of England's influence and growth of military power as well as tremendous developments in literature and science. Copernicus had revolutionized the way the planets and the relationship of the earth to the planets were viewed; Galileo's development of the telescope provided capabilities to view the stars and possibly answer all sorts of questions never dreamed possible. Those who pondered the nature of the cosmos in the classical period could do little beyond wonder, question, and construct elaborate arguments; Galileo, however, provided a means to actually see some elements of the universe, a feat not accomplished prior to his inventions. Faced with these amazing developments, it is no surprise that philosophy turned toward the ability to *see* things as an important focus for the development of knowledge.

PHILOSOPHY OF SIR FRANCIS BACON

The development of British empiricism took several forms. Locke, Berkeley, and Hume adopted a strictly philosophical approach; they explored the nature of knowledge and the operations of the mind and questioned crucial philosophical positions concerning causality and certainty. Though not considered one of the British Empiricists, Sir Francis Bacon contributed significantly to the movement. Bacon often is referred to as the "father of modern science" and the similarities in viewpoints among all these philosophers makes Bacon's contributions worth discussion as a part of the movement toward empiricism as the foundation for science. Bacon's emphasis on the development of a scientific method based on induction and experimentation is wholly consistent with the trends that have persisted in modern science. Nurses may find the following to be a particularly appealing aspect of Bacon's work: he strongly emphasized knowledge development activity not merely for the sake of scholarliness but as serving the public good.

BOX 4-1

FORMS OF EMPIRICISM

Empiricism exists in several forms, ranging from extreme to a more mild or weak position. Extreme or radical empiricism is the position that experience is the only source of knowledge; knowledge cannot be developed through any other means. A weak form of empiricism holds that sensory experience may be of some use in developing knowledge, but there is room for interpretation as to its specific value. Between these two positions is a moderate empiricism, which reflects the view that sensory experience does serve as a source of some knowledge. This position, however, does not exclude other possibilities as sources of knowledge generation.

Like the British Empiricists, Bacon lived and worked during the active time of Elizabethan England. Bacon was raised in a family with long ties to royalty and experienced a very privileged upbringing. At the influence of his family, particularly his father, Bacon developed a strong sense of duty to his country and to the service of humanity. He persisted in efforts to combine his interest in intellect and the workings of the human mind with his value for human service. Like Descartes, Bacon experienced a quality education but also developed a strong disdain for what was taught, for the standard texts and methods, and an overt hostility for the "cult" of Aristotle. Bacon's political and philosophical interests led to his commitment to set philosophy on a productive path away from mere scholastic argumentation to service toward promoting human good.

Emphasis on Applicable Knowledge

Bacon consistently wrote of his dedication to philosophy or more specifically to the mind itself. He aspired to be both a philosopher and a statesman; he believed that the focus of intellectual advancement should be on the application of knowledge for some practical purpose not on wisdom or on academic studies themselves. In one of his many essays, he clearly expressed his sentiment about excessive attention to study and the importance of the application of knowledge:

> To spend too much time in studies is sloth; to use them too much for ornament, is affectation; to make judgment wholly by their rules, is the humor of a scholar. They perfect nature, and are perfected by experience: for natural abilities are like natural plants that need pruning, by study; and studies themselves do give forth directions too much at large, except they be bounded in by experience. Crafty men condemn studies, simple men admire them, and wise men use them; for they teach not their own use; but that is a wisdom without them, and above them, won by observation. (Bacon, *Essays,* 1597/1995, p. 128)

Like Descartes, Bacon was struck by the errors, confusion, and lack of certainty evident in the philosophies and dogmas he had read and studied and that had influenced his schooling and life. Such teachings lacked confirmation and practical value due to the lack of application to nature. In a manner similar to Descartes, Bacon also sought a clean start to provide a new foundation that could lead to certainty and truth. Descartes turned to the mind as the source of knowledge; Bacon turned to nature with a goal of developing a means to generate practical and useful knowledge.

Bacon's emphasis on applying knowledge and developing useful knowledge marks an end to *Scholasticism*, which was characterized by the quest for knowledge for its own sake separate from observation and everyday use and reality. Scholasticism also showed a strong emphasis on debate and argumentation. Bacon instead emphasized experience rather than mere scholarly study and academic discourse.

Need for a New Method

As a statesman, Bacon was uniquely positioned to lead people to direct their attention to nature and observation when almost all emphasis had been focused elsewhere. His leadership role enabled him to advocate sweeping changes in the way knowledge was viewed and created while avoiding the hopelessness and skepticism that might have been associated with refuting existing ideas. Bacon shared with Descartes the belief that changes in method were needed to overcome the skepticism from previous attempts to develop knowledge of the world. Like Descartes, Bacon was thoroughly convinced that he possessed the ideas for a method that ultimately would provide a strong foundation for the discoveries that would make knowledge possible.

Bacon (1620/1939) began to express his views in the *Great Instauration*, which he intended to serve as a total redesign of science. In the *Prooemium* (Preface) to this work, Bacon (1620/1939) begins by describing in general the errors and difficulties that had confronted the "human intellect" and the effect of these errors on the development of human knowledge:

> Whence it follows that the entire fabric of human reason which we employ in the inquisition of nature is badly put together and built up, and like some magnificent structure without any foundation...there was but one course left, therefore—to try the whole thing anew upon a better plan, and to commence a total reconstruction of sciences, arts, and all human knowledge, raised upon the proper foundation. (pp. 5–6)

Bacon saw the essential task of the time to be the development of new methods and procedures that would aid the mind's intellectual capacities and allow it to operate to its fullest extent. He also desired to provide the philosophical foundation that would make such an activity appropriate. He never completed this work possibly because of the enormity of the task. It is equally likely that what Bacon had intended to accomplish was not totally plausible (Urbach, 1994, p. x). One of Bacon's most noteworthy works, however, comprised the second part of the Great Instauration and was titled the *Novum Organum* (1620/1994). The word *Organon*, derived from the Greek language, means *instrument*; Bacon saw his work as an instrument for setting science on the correct and fruitful path.

Embarking on this new method required first that people do away with existing assumptions, prejudices, and myths that influenced and ultimately obscured knowledge. Bacon described these prejudices as "Idols" and elaborated on four categories of idols: Idols of the Tribe, Cave, Marketplace, and Theater. Idols of the Tribe are related to human nature in general and arise from the "human spirit," "inadequacy of the senses," or human emotion (lii, p. 61).[1] The Idols of the Cave, or "Den" as they sometimes are called, refers to prejudices that result from the nature of an individual person—his or her unique mental and physical features, habits, and education[2] (liii, p. 61). Idols of the Marketplace "are the most troublesome of all" (lix, p. 64) and concern the influence of words and language on the quest for knowledge "for while men believe their reason governs words, in fact, words turn back and reflect their powers on the understanding, and so render philosophy and science sophistical and inactive" (lix, p. 64). Words also introduce "wrongness and error," and often are confused and poorly defined (lx, p. 41). Finally Bacon returns to an attack on previous philosophical positions; he describes the Idols of the Theater, which "are imposed and received entirely from the fictitious tales in theories, and from wrong-headed laws of demonstrations" (lxi, pp. 65–66). According to Bacon, these idols all pose significant barriers to the discovery of Truth and the development of science. Nurses should be able to identify examples of dogma and influences within the discipline and society at large that influence the continuing development of their knowledge base. Such examples are evident in the ways in which nursing is defined and differentiated from other disciplines, the accepted ways of teaching and practicing nursing, and modes of inquiry deemed suitable for nursing research.

In addition to the Idols, Bacon also saw other things that were wrong with philosophy and the "science" of the times and that had impeded progress to a great extent. First he saw philosophy as corrupted by logic, a criticism directly related to the demonstrations advocated by Aristotle. For Bacon, philosophy of this genre was oriented more to providing *an* answer than to discovering the inner truth of things (Bacon, lxiii, p. 68). While empiricists of Bacon's era did rely on data collection and on experimentation to some extent, they tended to function in the narrow realm of only a few experiments. According to Bacon, there was a pronounced tendency for "leap or flight to generalities and the principles of things" (Bacon, 1620/1994, lxiv,

---

[1]The *Novum Organum* is written as a series of aphorisms. In this chapter, roman numerals indicate the number of the aphorism. Page numbers are also provided to facilitate identifying the location of the material in the source referenced here.

[2]The reference to the *cave* is derived from Plato's well known allegory of the cave, presented in the *Dialogues*.

p. 70), arriving at sweeping conclusions that sometimes were far removed from their original data and experiments and, as a result, were likely to be far removed from the Truth as well. Superstition and theology also corrupted thinking and impeded progress for philosophers as well as for scientists (Bacon, 1620/1994, lxv, p.71).

Bacon cited additional reasons why science had not progressed at the time of his writing. Foremost among these was that science was not carried out in pursuit of the proper goal. According to Bacon (1620/1994), the "only true and proper goal of the sciences is to bring new discoveries and powers to human life" (lxxxi, p. 90). The work of scientists, as with the philosophers, showed a lingering reverence for authority and dogma including that imposed by the prevailing religion, government, and educational institutions. In addition to these significant restraints, scientists lacked reward for their work and they often functioned in isolation without any support for their inquiry. Equally important, scientists lacked even the proper method for study in the difficult context created by religious, social, and educational barriers to progress (lxxxii, pp. 90–92). Bacon argued that science was not conducted in a systematic manner with proper collection of data and thoughtful testing and observation. Instead scientists relied on tradition and argument "or the fluctuations and meanderings of chance and ambling and disorderly experience" (lxxxii, pp. 90–91). The results of scientific work, therefore, often reflected accident rather than meaningful discovery.

Therefore, science for all of its promise and possibilities had failed to accomplish anything trustworthy or meaningful for the human condition. Blinded by the prejudices gained through dogmatic teachings and encumbered by sociocultural barriers, scientists had much to overcome if their work was to be fruitful and useful. Finally Bacon pointed out that "but far the greatest obstacle to the progress of the sciences and the undertaking of new tasks and new fields lies in man's despair, and in his supposition that such advances are impossible" (xcii, p. 102). Bacon considered even the empirical school of philosophy to be fraught with error, giving rise to "more deformed and monstrous ideas than the *Sophistical* or rational" (lxiv, p. 70). This philosophy promoted conclusions based on the "narrow and obscure foundation of only a few experiments" (lxiv, p. 70) rather than on a broad and orderly search for Truth (lxx, p. 49). Proper method, however, could help to set science on a productive and hopeful path again.

Even if all of the other limitations somehow were overcome, Bacon argued that scientists lacked proper methods to conduct their inquiries. According to Bacon (1620/1994), the proper method of science involved experience "well-prepared and digested" (cii, p. 110), leading to the development of axioms as the early stages of the scientific process. Based on these axioms, new experiments could be conducted so that knowledge would be created in a systematic manner based on careful observation and analysis. For Bacon, this approach represented a closer league between experiment and reason with the detailed analysis of observations through experimentation. The fresh examination of the natural world (the particulars in the world) was to help science move beyond the accidental and disorderly discoveries of the past that prevented the attainment of knowledge.

The experiments that Bacon called for, however, were not to be conducted simply to discover causes and create axioms. Such actions would only be "experiments of light," or *experimenta lucifera*, to enlighten but possibly without any practical use. Instead Bacon called for *experimenta fructifera*, which would yield fruitful products, or knowledge that was useful. A different method of ordering and processing observations was needed to produce successful experiments (ic-c, p. 108–109).

Tables of Discovery

Bacon (1620/1994) created an elaborate scheme for organizing data that he referred to as the *Tables of Discovery*. The purpose of the Tables was to ensure that the scientist worked systematically and in a stepwise manner, moving from very specific axioms to somewhat broader or middle axioms and finally to the most general axioms. This would prevent the tendency to "leap and fly" from particulars to axiomatic statements, a tendency that Bacon argued was prevalent in much of the science taking place during his time. This schema of tables was oriented toward discovering the law or "form" that was the essential quality of every object. Like Plato, Bacon sought knowledge of Forms, the absolute essences. But these forms were to be found in nature not in the metaphysical realm apart from the reality of daily life.

Bacon explains how this is done in a detailed discussion of his three tables of investigation. First the investigator creates a Table of Affirmation based on "the rule of presence." For this table, the scientist compiles all known instances of a phenomenon that have the same characteristic. These instances are in agreement in form even though they may appear to be very dissimilar. Bacon was particularly interested in the study of heat with inquiry aimed at discovery of the nature or form of heat. The Table of Affirmation for the study of heat would include all instances in which heat is present such as in the sun's rays, lightning, flame, "hot" spices, human body fluids, even intense cold which bears some content of "heat."

The investigation proceeds to a Table of Negation, recording all instances in which the phenomenon (heat in this example) is totally absent. In the process of recording instances of Affirmation and Negation, Bacon points out that humans must recognize that our senses are not perfect. Scientists must be aided by experiments to overcome the potential for error in detecting presence and absence of a phenomenon because experiments make it possible to test observations regarding the presence or absence of the phenomenon.

When these two tables are completed, a process of comparison can be used to arrive at the nature of the phenomenon. In the example of heat, the tables reveal that heat cannot be weight because heavy objects could be found in both tables. A similar situation would be evident for other qualities of the instances listed in the tables. Through comparison of the tables, the scientist might determine that heat really is motion because motion is always present when heat is present and absent when heat is absent.

The process of scientific inquiry does not end at this point; according to Bacon, scientists need to verify further the results they have obtained. At this stage, a table of comparison is constructed to present instances in which the phenomenon is found to different extents ("the Table of Differing Degrees"). This table is used to demonstrate whether or not the former conclusion is correct. For example, if heat is motion, there should be more heat where there is more motion.

Bacon (1620/1994) acknowledged that merely filling in the tables might not be sufficient to generate meaningful results; he recognized that certain events or instances may warrant attention regardless of the effort that had taken place in regard to the Tables of Discovery. Bacon called these "prerogative instances," that is, cases by their very nature and singularity that demanded the scientist's attention. These instances represented situations so profound that the scientist could not avoid addressing them. Bacon identified no fewer then 27 categories of such instances to encompass a wide variety of attributes and characteristics. Overall the attention that Bacon gave to such instances that might be missed in the completion of the Tables reveals the importance of a thorough and comprehensive approach to induction and organization of data in Bacon's method.

Implications

Bacon's writings on science are significant in a number of ways. Bacon's work is not significant for any contributions to developing empiricism within western epistemology. Bacon did not address, for example, the role of the senses in the development of knowledge, discussion that is critical in empiricist thought. Bacon did, however, present other messages that have contributed to an enduring legacy. These messages have considerable relevance for contemporary scientists and for nurse scholars as well.

Bacon presented striking arguments against dogma and authority and pointedly called attention to the role of tradition in impeding productive activity. This observation presents a situation familiar to nurses. Nursing has numerous examples of dogmatic thinking including reference to nursing as caring, an art and science, and nursing process. Similarly many nursing practices are carried out because of tradition rather than any sound base of evidence or research. In response to the situations he observed, Bacon promoted systematic and rigorous inquiry with close attention to detail as the foundation of proper scientific method. This idea of rigor and systematic method continues to be a hallmark of science and quality inquiry centuries later.

Bacon's work as a statesman has a particularly compelling aspect for nurses. Bacon adamantly called for fruitful inquiry aimed to serve the public good. There is a clear contrast with many other philosophies in which there is a presumption that knowledge alone is a sufficient and appropriate goal. For Bacon, however, the properly placed goal of science is conducted to improve human life, providing "new discoveries and powers" (Bacon, 1620/1994, lxxxi, p. 90). This practical end for inquiry is particularly fitting for nurses who strive to improve human existence through their science. Bacon admonished his readers not to despair at the lack of progress in science prior to his writings. Nurses might benefit as well from Bacon's lesson of hope for pursuit of answers through relief from dogma and tradition.

IDEAS OF JOHN LOCKE

As seen in the previous discussion of the work of Sir Francis Bacon, the 17th century in western epistemology was marked by an emphasis on empiricism, or experience as the basis for knowledge. Empiricism can take many forms; some strictly emphasize experience and others present a relatively weak emphasis. In its weakest sense, empiricism is the doctrine that our senses provide us with some form of *knowledge*. This form of empiricism can be generalized into the argument that *all* knowledge comes from experience in some way; it allows the possibility that experience is a stimulus or originator of knowledge but there is room for other elements beyond that. In an extreme form, empiricism claims that no source other than experience provides knowledge at all. Plato and Descartes provide examples of arguments against such a view with the ideology that the world of sensory data is so changeable and the senses so fallible, that knowledge cannot possibly be acquired through sensory data.

The writings of John Locke present a stark contrast to these earlier philosophies because Locke argues for a stricter empiricist view of knowledge. Locke produced a number of significant works in his lifetime and is known in many sectors for his *Two Treatises of Government* (1689/1967), a highly influential work of political philosophy. However, in epistemology, Locke gave empiricism a foothold in British philosophy, providing a foundation later built upon by George Berkeley (1965)[1] and the Scottish philosopher David Hume (1748/1975, 1740/1978). Locke's (1690/1975) *Essay Concerning Human Understanding*[2] represents a prominent contribution to empiricism as the basis for knowledge and provides much of the philosophical foundation that undergirds the development of modern science.

Origins of Knowledge

The stimulus for the *Essay* mirrors much of the lingering debate about the origins of knowledge. In the beginning of the *Essay* in a section titled Epistle to the Reader (1690/1975), Locke describes how some friends meeting in his "chambers" became stymied by difficulties that arose in the course of their conversation. Locke proposed that before they could inquire further, "it was necessary to examine our own abilities and see what objects our understanding were, or were

---

[1]In very simple terms, Berkeley, the Irish philosopher, took Locke's emphasis on ideas and argued that ideas actually were objects presented to the senses. Berkeley objected to the notion of an "abstract idea" since such an entity would rely on imagination. According to Berkeley, it would not be possible to imagine "rectangle" or "color" without reference to actual rectangles or items possessing specific colors. Berkeley argued that nothing can exist outside of perception, and physical objects thus are comprised of sensations and ideas; things exist only as they are perceived.

[2]Hereafter referred to as the *Essay*.

not, fitted to deal with" (p. 7). This conversation with his friends started Locke on the inquiries that continued intermittently for approximately 20 years.

Similar to Bacon, Descartes' works held a particularly important and influential position for Locke. This influence is apparent immediately in the *Essay* because Locke (1690/1975) devoted the whole of the first book of the *Essay* to an elaborate (some readers might say "excessive") criticism and refutation of one of Descartes' central doctrines, the doctrine of innate ideas. Locke posed several reasons why this doctrine was not acceptable. First, according to Locke, the existence of innate ideas is not self-evident; the fact that there may be general agreement about their existence does not make their existence a reality. Second, if there were innate ideas, there should be principles to which every human subscribes. Locke argued, however, that there were many ideas not known to children, "idiots," and a substantial portion of humankind. Consequently there must not be any universality to the ideas that the mind is supposed to possess. Finally Locke argued that it was impossible for some principle to be innate yet for the mind to not perceive its presence. For example, if *pain* were an innate idea, the mind should be aware of its existence. Locke conceded that humans have natural faculties or capacities to think and reason. That is not the same as having innate ideas. This rejection of innate ideas makes it possible for Locke to propose the notion of the mind as "white paper, void of all characters, without any Ideas" (Bk. II, chap. I, sect. 2, p. 104), or as a "blank slate" or **tabula rasa**, in common terms (although Locke did not use this specific phrase).

Locke then is faced with the challenge to argue from where knowledge does originate, if it does not originate from innate ideas. Locke's (1690/1975) unequivocal answer is that all knowledge originates *from experience;* experience produces the ideas that are essential for human thought (Bk. II, chap. I, sect. 2, p. 104). Locke's notion of idea is as an object of thought not as something innate, as Descartes had argued. An **idea**, for Locke, is "the object of understanding when a man [sic] thinks...whatever it is, which the mind can be employed about in thinking" (p. 47). This definition of *idea* is one of the central notions of Locke's *Essay*.

Having stipulated that notion of idea, Locke formulated a second central theme of the *Essay*, which concerns the essence of the mind. Again responding to the work of Descartes, Locke argued that the essence of the mind cannot be to think, as Descartes had proposed. If the essence of the mind were to think, the mind could not exist and not be thinking; some ideas (as Locke defined them) would have to be innate since, according to Locke, ideas are the objects of thought. Locke already had argued against this notion of innate ideas. The remaining possibility for the essence of the mind to be thinking indicated that, in the absence of innate ideas, the mind could exist only after experience furnished it with ideas. This was not an acceptable position either because it was reasonable to believe that the mind existed prior to experience. If not, how could the mind take in experience and formulate any ideas?

Nature of Experience

Locke (1690/1975) refuted two primary themes in Descartes epistemology; he argued against the doctrine of innate ideas and Descartes' position that the essence of the mind was to think. Locke proposed instead that the mind essentially was the same as a blank sheet of paper before any ideas were present and that it existed as the capacity to receive ideas. According to Locke, a person first begins to think "when he first has any sensation" (Bk. II, chap. I, sect. 23).

On first reading, the importance of the above argument in regard to the development of modern philosophy and particularly modern science could easily be overlooked; yet the impact of this philosophical view was quite profound. Locke's contribution to the subsequent development of science stems to a great extent from his argument that all ideas, hence all *knowledge*, come from experience. This principle provides the foundation for the empiricism that has directed the development of science since Locke's time because science has been focused on data gathered through sensory experience as the basis for the development of scientific knowledge.

Experience, according to Locke (1690/1975), was not limited to sensation alone. Actually Locke identified two types of experience that would lead to ideas in the mind. The experience of **sensation** occurred when the senses were affected by something external, such as an external physical object, thereby leading to the creation of ideas such as yellow, green, hot, cold, soft, and bitter. Experience, however, also included more internal processes that Locke called **reflection**. Reflection involved examination of the operations of the person's own mind. Through reflection, the individual would experience processes such as perceiving, thinking, doubting, believing, reasoning, willing, and knowing.

Formation of Complex Ideas

Experience derived from either sensation or reflection generates in the mind a **simple idea**, which Locke defined as "one uniform appearance or conception in the mind, and is not distinguishable into different ideas" (Bk. I, chap. II, sect. 1, p. 119). Once the mind had been furnished with a number of simple ideas, the mind had the power to compare, repeat, or join those ideas in an almost infinite variety of combinations. Although the mind took on an active role at this stage to form **complex ideas**, Locke was clear in describing how the mind passively received the simple ideas that formed the original foundation for knowledge (Bk. I, chap. I, sect. 23, p. 118).

In constructing the complex ideas, the mind compares, contrasts, and joins simple ideas according to a variety of criteria. Locke identified specifically the processes that occur in the mind in the framing of complex ideas. Simple ideas can be combined directly into one compound or complex idea, the basis for the development of all complex ideas. There are other complex ideas, however, that

Locke addressed as ideas of Relation and Abstraction; these are developed through the careful examination of and comparison among a number of simple ideas (Bk. II, chap. XII, p. 163).

Locke's (1690/1975) discussion of the mind as having an active role in the development of complex ideas seems to introduce an element of rationalism into Locke's foundation of empiricism. This is precisely the element he intended to avoid. Even with the mind having this role, it is clear that the original source of all knowledge is the simple ideas derived from experience. The origin of knowledge, therefore, is experience and not the innate content or the workings of the mind. Perhaps even more important is Locke's position that the mind cannot form complex ideas arbitrarily. All these complex ideas are still true to their original source, the simple ideas, because "of these the mind can have no more, nor other than what are suggested to it" (Bk II, ch XII, sect. 2, p. 164).

Locke's argument results in the position that the complex ideas have an objective reality; this is in contrast to claims of possible subjectivity that might be levied against a purely rational (based on reason) approach to knowledge. Some philosophers credit concepts with some *a priori* (prior to experience) component beyond a strictly empirical origin rather than being the objects of sensory experience.[1] Locke, however, viewed concepts in a manner consistent with an underlying **physical realism**: that there is an objective reality with distinct *things* or objects in it and that it is possible to receive or construct ideas that mirror that reality. The idea of the mind as a "mirror" of reality can be found in many philosophical discussions of knowledge.

The consistent theme throughout Locke's *Essay* is that the ideas that people hold represent real things existing outside the person. These ideas constitute the link by which knowledge of the external physical world is developed. The metaphor of the mind as a mirror of reality is often used to reflect this relationship of physical reality and ideas. According to Locke's description, the mind is capable of reflecting only what is set before it; this representation of physical reality can be assumed to be clear and accurate because the mind serves only to reflect reality or to form concepts based on the ideas generated through mirroring the physical world.

Development of Knowledge from Ideas

In the final section of the *Essay* (the fourth book), Locke explains in detail how ideas become *knowledge*. Knowledge in general is the perception of the connection and agreement or disagreement of ideas (Bk. IV, chap. I, sect. 2, p. 525). Knowledge does not extend beyond the ideas, especially the connections and agree-

---

[1]See Kant, I. (1929), *Critique of pure reason*, who describes concepts as "rules" that exist naturally in the mind and that, consequently, make experience possible; see chapter 5.

ments among ideas. Different types, or degrees, of knowledge relate to how the perception of agreement or disagreement occurs: intuition, demonstration, and sensitive knowledge. Intuition consists of the perception of agreement or disagreement of two ideas immediately and by themselves without intervention of any other ideas. This immediate perception leaves no room for doubt or hesitation and contributes to certainty in perceptions (Bk. IV, chap. II, sect. 4, p. 531).

Demonstration is another form of knowledge described by Locke (1690/1975) in which intervening ideas in the form of proofs are introduced to the mind. In other words, proofs show (demonstrate) the connection of ideas through intermediate ideas to from knowledge. There is progression to arrive at the conclusion through an incremental process (Bk. IV, chap. II, sect. 4, p. 532) much as a logical argument is constructed. The process is much like the way in which theorems and proofs are presented in geometry. Demonstrative knowledge, according to Locke, has a high degree of certainty because the intermediate proofs serve to address areas of potential doubt and so remove this doubt from the resulting knowledge.

Finally sensitive knowledge is "employed about the particular existence of finite beings without us, which going beyond bare probability and yet not reaching perfectly to either of the foregoing degrees of certainty, passes under the name of knowledge" (Bk. IV, chap. II, sect. 14, p. 537). In other words, sensitive knowledge is focused on objects in the external world. This knowledge is not just circumstantial, that is, clouded by the fallibility of sensation; yet it also produces less certainty than either intuition or demonstration.

In summary, Locke's position on knowledge begins with a focus on the mind that at birth is essentially a "blank slate." Although initially devoid of ideas, the mind possesses a universal capacity to *receive* ideas. As a person experiences the world (external reality) through sensation (or as the mind reflects on its own activity), simple ideas result in the mind. These simple ideas can combine to form complex ideas. The use of reason to determine the agreement or disagreement among ideas results in knowledge. As the mind becomes familiar with ideas, it remembers and gives names to them. Ideas, words, and the use of reason grow together and assent to the truth of propositions (statements about the world).

Consistent with an empirical approach, Locke placed emphasis in discussions of knowledge on the relationship between experience and knowledge. For Locke, ideas in the mind were derived directly through the experiences of sensation and reflection; ideas are representations of either the physical world or of the processes of the mind.

This approach, however, seems to reduce knowledge to mere mental images. According to this view, knowledge resides in the mind in the form of ideas and it is not possible for others to see or verify these ideas. Even though the ideas result from experience, knowledge comes from ideas and from the perception of connection and agreement among ideas. Consequently it would seem necessary to peer inside someone's mind to determine what knowledge he or she possessed. The ability to reexamine the processes by which someone formulated the ideas and resulting knowledge would be of even greater value.

DAVID HUME'S EXPANSION OF LOCKE'S WORK

David Hume, a Scottish philosopher and a contributor to British empiricism, made a tighter connection between experience and knowledge, thus offering an important extension of Locke's work. Consistent with Locke's views and essential to an empiricist philosophy, Hume clearly disputed Descartes' position regarding the existence of any "innate ideas;" he argued instead that all mental content was derived from experience. Hume produced two pivotal works, *A Treatise of Human Nature*[1] (Hume, 1740/1978), which is subtitled *An Attempt to Introduce the Experimental Method of Reasoning into Moral Subjects,* and *An Enquiry Concerning Human Understanding* (Hume, 1748/1975). Hume desired to provide a method to overcome the nonrational aspects of human nature through the use of experimental method (Jacobson, 1996). Human nature, which is imperfect and prone to error, needed the direction provided by experiment, deducing "general principles from a comparison of particular instances." Hume presented this procedure in stark contrast to the previously popular approaches in which broad principles first were established with specific conclusions developed subsequently from those principles. For Hume, this latter process produced only mistake and illusion (Hume, 1748/1975, p. 174).

Expanding on Locke's views, Hume (1740/1978) began his *Treatise* with the following statement: "All the perceptions of the human mind resolve themselves into two distinct kinds, which I shall call ***impressions*** and ***ideas***" (Bk. I, part I, sect. i, p.1). With this viewpoint, Hume distinguished between the processes of sensing and thinking. Impressions result from perceptions and are derived from actual experience (sensing). For example, a person can feel the cold when walking through snowy countryside. A person also can think about being cold. Such thinking produces an *idea* of cold. While these outcomes may seem quite similar to the person doing the sensing or thinking, Hume theorized that the results in the mind are quite different, particularly in their intensity. Impressions carry significantly more impact and vividness, and are more intense than is characteristic of similar ideas. This distinction between sensing and thinking sometimes is referred to as Hume's fork.[2]

Hume (1740/1978) included both sensation and reflection as elements of the perception that produces impressions. This position represents a significant addi-

---

[1]Hereafter referred to as the *Treatise.*

[2]Hume's fork, more specifically, refers to the distinction between matters of fact and relations of ideas. Similar metaphors are used in regard to the positions of a number of philosophers, one of the more familiar ones being Ockham's razor, which refers generally to simplicity and belief in the smallest possible number of types of objects, or the least possible factors in presenting an argument. In regard to Hume, the metaphor of fork vividly captures the nature of a specific dichotomy such as Hume's distinction between sensing and thinking.

tion to Locke's works, which only identified sensation and reflection as aspects of experience. Hume instead went a step further in identifying impressions as the result of both sensation and reflection and adding memory and imagination as the source of ideas. As elements of reflection, Hume included passions, desires, and emotions—things that can be perceived by the individual. Hume further refined Locke's scheme regarding the relationship between experience and ideas and directly addressed memory and imagination as significant mental activities. Impressions and ideas bear a close resemblance except in their "degree of force and vivacity...so that all the perceptions of the mind are double, and appear both as impressions and ideas" (pp. 2–3). Hume placed limits on the implications of this position by making use of Locke's distinction between *simple* and *complex* ideas. Simple impressions and ideas cannot be divided into smaller components; complex ideas, in contrast, can be divided into parts. As an example, Hume describes an apple, which can be divided into qualities of color, taste, and smell (Bk. I, part I, sect. i, p. 2). This notion of simple and complex is useful to explain why some ideas and impressions do not relate to each other ("are not resembling") (p. 3); in other words, the mind can possess an idea of something for which it has no direct, related impression. This is possible because complex ideas are formed from the simple ones. A complex idea may not have an impression directly related to it. Simple ideas and simple impressions, however, do resemble each other (p. 4). According to Hume's arguments, they are in fact directly connected: "All our simple ideas proceed either mediately or immediately, from their correspondent impressions... This, then, is the first principle I establish in the science of human nature; nor ought we to despise it because of the simplicity of its appearance" (p. 7). Hume attempted to "restore the word *idea* to its original sense, from which Mr. Locke had perverted it in making it stand for all our perceptions" (p. 2, footnote). For Hume, impressions are the perceptions themselves and ideas are the objects of the mind.

Functions of the Mind

For Hume (1748/1975), the mind is passive in the formation of impressions. Still the mind has some creative powers. The mind, for example, can distinguish simple ideas and reunite them in "what form it pleases" (p. 10). This acknowledgment explains how the mind constructs ideas such as that of the unicorn; although such a creature cannot be experienced in real life, the mind can possess an idea of such a being. Such processes do not occur arbitrarily, however, and it is easy to imagine the resulting chaos and the high degree of subjectivity if the mind acted so freely. As Hume stated, "nothing would be more unaccountable than the operations of that faculty were it not guided by some universal principles, which render it, in some measure, uniform with itself in all times and places" (p. 10). Clearly the connection of ideas cannot be left to chance. Hume argues that some universal principles exist to guide this mental process, and identifies three qualities that aid in this mental function: *Resemblance, Contiguity* in time or place, and *Cause and Effect.*

Hume believed that it is not necessary to provide a detailed account of how these qualities make it possible to determine an association among ideas. Indeed it is easy to see how two ideas that resemble each other could be associated in the mind without difficulty. This situation also holds for ideas related in time and space. The quality of cause and effect, however, warrants further discussion and occupies a considerable portion of both the *Treatise* and the *Enquiry*.

Relations identified through resemblance and contiguity in time and space force the mind to adhere to what is immediately present. In other words, the mind cannot leap beyond what is present to it to determine these associations. Determination of causation, however, presents quite the opposite situation:

> Here then it appears, that of those three relations, which depend not upon the mere ideas, the only one, that can be trac'd beyond our senses, and informs us of existences and objects, which we do not see or feel, is *causation*. (Bk I, part II, sect. 3, p. 74)

In discussing causation, Hume's ideas are based on the radical position that people are ruled by custom and instinct in the most important aspects of human existence. Cause, which occupied such a pivotal position in Aristotle's philosophy (where the *cause* of a thing's existence was its *essence*), for Hume is a matter of custom or habit. To understand this position in regard to its implications for knowledge, Hume proceeds to distinguish three kinds of human reason: *Knowledge, proofs,* and *probabilities.* **Knowledge** is based on the comparison of ideas, whereas **proofs** are "those arguments, which are deriv'd from the relation of cause and effect, and which are entirely free from doubt and uncertainty" (Bk. I, part XI, sect. 3, p. 124). Proofs are particularly well substantiated and go beyond mere probability, which still involves a degree of uncertainty. For Hume, "all our reasonings concerning the probability of causes are founded on the transferring of past to future" (p. 137). **Probability**, therefore, is based simply on habit, that is, derived from expectations created through prior experience.

In making this position about probability and in subsequent discussion of the similar notion of necessary connections, Hume attempts to set aside much of earlier epistemology, thereby giving further credibility to his empiricist position. Ultimately Hume works toward the position "that all our reasonings concerning causes and effects are derived from nothing but custom; and that belief is more properly an act of the sensitive, than of the cogitative part of our natures (Bk. I, part I, sect. 4, p. 183). Quantity, however, involves precise standards, making it possible to determine quantity relations "without any possibility of error" (Bk. I, part I, sect. 3, p. 71). Hume, interestingly, sees these rules as applying only to algebra and arithmetic "as the only sciences in which we can carry on a chain of reasoning to any degree of intricacy, and yet preserve a perfect exactness and certainty" (p. 71). Hume regards geometry as far less perfect because its fundamental principles are based on appearances such as shapes and proportions.

Hume made a substantial contribution to the empiricist tradition by adding clarity to Locke's thesis and further institutionalizing the notion that "knowledge" consists of that which cannot be false. Hume expressed regret that this work had not gained more attention and notoriety; yet it was noted widely for containing a hint of skepticism that often led to a negative response to his work. His biographer, Mossner (1980), commented that "the *Treatise* was sufficiently alive in 1745 to lose for Hume the Professorship of Ethics and Pneumatical Philosophy at Edinburgh" (p. 117). While debate continues about the degree of skepticism inherent in his work (Fogelin, 1985; Wright, 1983), Hume's position on knowledge and the role of custom or instinct in human existence has left an indelible mark on epistemology.

 ## CONCLUSION

Locke, as well as Hume and many of their contemporaries, also wrote on moral and political philosophy. In fact, many people are familiar with Locke primarily because of his renowned writings on government and politics. Hume similarly created several works concerning these other branches of philosophy. One entire Book of the work, *A Treatise of Human Nature* (1740/1978) is titled "Of Morals." Rather than view these as separate areas of inquiry it is easy to see how epistemology and political and moral philosophy are closely intertwined. Epistemology, the study of knowledge, is not easily separated from discussions of human nature, will, reason, life, and liberty. This is an important observation that may not be recognized by apparent focusing on their views of knowledge alone. Yet it is worth considering and is perhaps a weakness in more contemporary (i.e., Modern) philosophies of science that were to come centuries later and that overlooked the important role of the human in discussions of knowledge and science. Actually the early philosophers of science did not overlook the human aspect; they found it totally inappropriate to discussions of science, thus human behavior had no role in the development of science.[1]

For epistemology, the tradition of the British Empiricists laid the foundation for the entire "modern" period of thinking on knowledge and science. They clung to a belief in absolutes and truth and attempted to justify these beliefs by examining the workings of the human mind. The mind ultimately was the vehicle for sorting and organizing ideas and impressions. Truth, or real knowledge, was derived from experience particularly of the objects of the world. This focus on external reality ultimately served as the foundation for modern science that has dominated western societies in their attempts to understand the world of existence and is the focal point of the majority of traditional research methods.

---

[1]See, for example, Schlick's famous reference to ethics as mere emotion. See also chapter 6.

Nursing practice and research show the influence of empiricism. Sensory data necessarily play an important role in nursing practice and include a variety of visual cues and physiologic measures. Nursing research also has shown a strong history of the use of observational tools for data collection. A question that persists for nurses, however, concerns the potential existence of other forms of data that enable nurses to move beyond what they see and hear to access parts of human existence that are not empirical in nature such as dignity, personhood, hope, or grief.

In spite of these concerns in nursing, there is no question that the philosophical tradition known as British empiricism has had a profound impact on the development of science and research methods. This group of philosophers emphasized the external, physical world as the objects of knowledge and the role of the senses in gaining that knowledge. The inner workings of the mind may have a role in constructing that knowledge, but the focus is on external elements that are the source of that knowledge. It is most important that the knowledge matches the external world and is consistent with physical reality.

The metaphor of the mind as a "mirror" provides a good illustration of the importance of accurately reflecting the physical world. These empiricists did not address many elements such as generalizability and control that have become part of current understanding of quality science. It is clear, however, that the empiricists would focus further knowledge work on the physical world and gaining clear and accurate representations of the world (i.e., objective). This foundation certainly contributed to later developments in both philosophy and methodology in science.

Such views created numerous problems, however, with one of the most prominent for nurses concerning the role of subjective, personal experience. For the empiricists, such experience would have to be rendered somehow in a form that could be perceived by the senses. While it might be possible to have knowledge of facial expressions or body movements, would it be possible to have "knowledge" of happiness, comfort, dignity, or suffering? For the empiricists, such elements of human existence were not the focus of knowledge. Modern scientists have needed to create means to have knowledge of such things particularly through the development of instruments to measure and objectify human feeling. Sensory data alone seems to capture only part of the picture of human experience. The Empiricists' challenge to nurses (and others) is how to capture things that cannot be seen or touched. If the view of humans as complex, sentient beings with emotions and unique individual histories is at all correct, it is essential that nurses understand the varied aspects of human existence.

 ## FOR DISCUSSION

1. Although it is difficult to imagine, consider the possibility of a person who lacked any sensory ability—no sight, taste, smell, hearing, touch. If the individual were born without these abilities, could this person have any knowledge?

How would an empiricist such as Locke answer this question? How do you think Descartes would respond?

2. How would your response to the above questions change if the person had been born with some sensory ability but later lost that sensation or had only one or two functioning senses?

3. Discuss examples of the use of empirical and nonempirical inquiry in nursing research and practice.

4. Consider examples of phenomena that are not usually thought of as empirical but that are studied in an empirical manner. A few examples include phenomena such as hope, justice, dignity, and spirituality. What are the advantages and limitations of such an approach to inquiry, both for the research and for the discipline of nursing?

REFERENCES

Bacon, F. (1939). The great instauration, Prooemium. In E. A. Burtt (Ed.), *The English philosophers from Bacon to Mill* (pp. 5–23). New York: Random House. (Original work published 1620).

Bacon, F. (1994). *Novum Organum.* (P. Urbach and J. Gibson, Trans. and Ed.). Chicago: Open Court. (Original work published 1620).

Bacon, F. (1995). Of studies. In F. Bacon, *Essays* (pp. 128–129). New York: Prometheus Books. (Original work published 1597).

Berkeley, G. (1965). *Berkeley's philosophical writings* (D. M. Armstrong, Ed.). London: Collier.

Fogelin, R. J. (1985). *Hume's skepticism in the treatise of human nature.* London: Routledge & Kegan Paul.

Hume, D. (1975). *An enquiry concerning human understanding and an enquiry concerning the principles of morals* (L. A. Selby-Bigge, Ed., 3rd rev. ed., P. H. Nidditch, Ed.). Oxford: Oxford University Press. (Original work published 1748).

Hume, D. (1978). *A treatise of human nature,* (L. A. Selby-Bigge, Ed. 2nd rev. ed., P. Nidditch, Ed.). Oxford: Oxford University Press. (Original work published 1740).

Jacobson, A. J. (1996). David Hume on human understanding. In S. Brown, (Ed.), *British philosophy and the age of enlightenment* (pp. 150–178).

Locke, J. (1967). *Two treatises of government* (2nd Ed.). (P. Laslett, Ed.). Cambridge: Cambridge University Press. (Original work published 1689).

Locke, J. (1975). *An essay concerning human understanding* (P. Nidditch, Ed.). Oxford: Oxford University Press. (Original work published 1690).

Mossner, E. C. (1980). *The life of David Hume* (2nd ed.). Oxford: Clarendon Press.

Urbach, P. (1994). Editor's introduction. In P. Urbach and J. Gibson (Trans. and Ed.), *Francis Bacon: Novum Organum* (pp. ix–xxvii). Chicago: Open Court.

Wright, J. P. (1983). *The sceptical realism of David Hume.* Minneapolis, MN: University of Minnesota Press.

CHAPTER 5

The Transcendental Idealism of Immanuel Kant

KEY IDEAS

analytic	nursing knowledge
a priori	nursing science
categories	objective
concepts	phenomena
epistemology	sensibility
Hume's fork	space
idealism	subject-predicate form
intuition	subjective
knowledge	synthetic
metaphysics	time
noumena	

One pervasive question about nursing knowledge concerns the relationship between the knowledge base of the discipline and "science." The traditional view of science is derived from the foundation provided by the British Empiricists, where science is based on what is observed or otherwise perceived through the senses. A considerable portion of the knowledge used in nursing fits that description without difficulty. All of the basic science content important in nursing, such as chemistry, microbiology, and information related to disease and pharmacologic agents, is consistent with an empirical focus. Nurses gain keen skills to observe, auscultate, and palpate as a part of their education and in a large number of practice settings. This critical information in nursing easily can be thought of as "science."

However, a substantial part of nursing, including much of what seems to set nursing apart from other disciplines, does not fit the usual mold of science. Important concepts such as *hope, spirituality, empathy, presence,* and *caring* to name just a few cannot be understood through empirical means alone. This aspect of nursing typically is referred to as the "art" of nursing in contrast to the "science."

Of course, there have been many efforts to make some parts of this nonempirical realm of nursing fit with science and become recognized as legitimate bodies of scientific knowledge. Numerous programs of research have led to useful means to measure seemingly nonempirical entities such as coping, quality of life, and grief. Success has been varied in the effort to make abstract entities fit the mold of science, however, with grief serving as a particularly prominent example. For many years, work to develop an effective tool for observing (measuring) grief did not progress beyond essentially a checklist of symptoms. Although instruments for abstract phenomena such as grief, coping, and stress do exist, the question remains whether or not such an approach to inquiry is the most effective way to understand these human experiences.

Such results leave nursing with several options. Nurses can continue to try and force such things into the traditional mold of empiricism and to continue work on making such phenomena observable. If this can be accomplished, nursing could be legitimized as a "science" consistent with other traditional sciences. Whatever cannot fit this idea of science can be considered the "art" of nursing or in some cases may be disregarded as irrelevant because of the nonscientific nature of such phenomena.

This scenario has been pursued in regard to many phenomena of interest to nurses; remnants of this argument about legitimizing nursing science can be found in a number of discussions about nursing knowledge. Several ways of conceptualizing nursing knowledge are apparent in the literature; they mirror this tension between science, empiricism, and other forms of knowledge. These are presented in Box 5-1 in statements reflecting the relationship between nursing knowledge, broadly defined, and "science." These statements demonstrate some ways in which the nursing knowledge base can be described.

As Box 5-1 demonstrates, options are available for descriptions of nursing knowledge that do not require an empirical approach to significant phenomena. Empiricism has attained a position of high status as a form of knowledge in western societies. It is not, however, the only form of knowledge that exists. Perhaps part of nursing is empirical, but other equally important portions are nonempirical in nature. **Nursing knowledge** may be broader than **nursing science**. In other words, nursing knowledge could be thought of as comprised of "science" (empiricism) along with something else. Nurses probably are very comfortable with this idea, and the *something else* typically has been described as "art." Unfortunately this has created a false dichotomy between art and science. An alternative would

BOX 5-1

DEFINITIONS OF NURSING KNOWLEDGE

1. Nursing knowledge = Science, and Science = Empiricism.
2. Nursing knowledge = Science (Empiricism) + X
3. Nursing knowledge = Science, and Science is > Empiricism
4. Nursing knowledge ≠ Science

be to think of the "something else" as a legitimate form of knowledge. This raises a new question for consideration, particularly in view of the high status given to empiricism: How is it possible to have credible knowledge that is nonempirical in nature?

◆ KANT'S *CRITIQUE OF PURE REASON*

This is, to some extent, similar to the type of dilemma confronted by Kant 1781/1965) in his *Critique of Pure Reason*. While writing this work, rationalism and religion heavily influenced thought in Kant's native Prussia and much of Europe. Reason had become the focus of much discussion about knowledge. In the sphere of metaphysics, remarkable claims were being made that were defended only by reason. The existence of God, for example, and the nature of the human spirit or free will were nonempirical knowledge claims defended only by strong arguments based on reason. Arguments that had been advanced and supported by reason usually fell apart; in other words, reason alone had been insufficient to support a number of important claims. Without reason, however, religion seemed threatened. The fact that no one had seen heaven through a telescope posed a serious threat to the role of religion and religious authority.

Even science was in danger as a result of Hume's skepticism. By reducing causal connections to custom or habit and doing away with the idea of necessary connections while focusing on probability, even scientific knowledge seemed impossible. Kant aimed to save both religion and science: to show reason not as the source of ultimate truth about the world but to show what it could accomplish and to save science from skepticism by supplying the elements of necessity and universality required by scientific knowledge.

Kant's approach was to look at knowledge in a different way with the possibility of combining experience and reason. Kant agreed with many of his predecessors that experience does not furnish anything more than probability and is only partial evidence of what occurs before our eyes. No number of experiences can provide complete proof that things always follow the same pattern or that the same sequence of events takes place universally.

For Kant, knowledge entails elements of certainty: it is necessary and universal. Aristotle, Descartes, and others all pointed out the limitations of sensory experience alone in determining what is necessary and universal. Kant, like Descartes, is interested in the capabilities of reason, that is, the power of reason apart from experience. The main question pursued in the *Critique of Pure Reason* is how much can be known through understanding and reason apart from experience?

A *Priori* Judgments

Kant (1781/1965) substitutes a more philosophical question: "How are synthetic *a priori* judgments possible?" (p. 55). In other words, how is it possible to make connections among things and have the result seem credible as "knowledge" in the absence of experience to support those connections? The phrase *a priori* captures the reference to being apart from experience, in other words, *prior to* experience. Experience does not meet the criteria of being necessary or universal; some *a priori* element, however, would have to be essential and valid for everyone simply because it is not tied to the dynamic and highly contextualized realm of experience. The term **synthetic** refers to a connection.

Kant considered this problem of the possibility of synthetic *a priori* judgments to be the crucial concern of **metaphysics** as evident in the following passage: "Upon the solution of this problem, or upon a sufficient proof that the possibility which it desires to have explained does in fact not exist at all, depends the success or failure of metaphysics" (Kant, 1781/1965, p. 55). Kant dismissed Hume's work, which had been focused on synthetic statements and particularly the connection of cause and effect. Kant considered the skeptic Hume to have been on a path leading to the "destruction of all pure philosophy"[1] (p. 55). According to Kant's (1783/1902) discussion in the *Prolegomena*, one important shortcoming of Hume's work was that he considered mathematical statements to be analytic. In contrast, Kant took the position that mathematical statements are synthetic. If Kant could support his case that mathematics was in fact synthetic then he could demonstrate that *a priori* synthetic judgments were possible. Mathematics is an excellent case for such argument as it lacks any empirical correlates. It is possible to see 7 oranges or 5 cats or 11 nurses but it is not possible to see the numbers themselves. In other words, numbers alone cannot be experienced using the senses; only their application is sensory.

Analytic judgments based on experience are commonplace. It is a simple matter, for example, to break apart a chemical compound to identify its constituent components. Similarly we can observe how the synthesis of two chemical elements

---

[1]Pure philosophy, the term commonly applied to Metaphysics, generally is regarded as the study of the nature of reality.

produces a new compound. But how do we use reason alone to combine or synthesize things outside of experience to produce something new? Mathematics provides an excellent example of how such *a priori* synthetic judgments are used all the time. For example, 7 and 5 can be combined to produce 12; this is a wholly synthetic statement. An analytic approach would be to take the number 12, break it apart, and expect to find 7 and 5. Yet this is not possible. Laws of physics work the same way. We cannot analytically determine by picking matter apart that it is neither created nor destroyed. The property of being "neither created nor destroyed" is not *in* matter just as 5 and 7 are not *in* 12. We can say such things, for example, about math and about matter—we can *know* these things—without any validation through experience.

The distinction between analytic and synthetic judgments can be considered an elaborate form of what is sometimes referred to as "Hume's Fork." Hume divided all propositions into those that express relations of ideas (analytic) and those that express matters of fact (synthetic). Rather than focus on ideas and facts as the basis for distinguishing analytic and synthetic, Kant (1965) tied his arguments to a discussion of the grammatical **subject-predicate form**. Analytic judgments exist in situations where a predicate (something that can be predicated of a subject) already exists in the subject:

> Either the predicate to the subject A, as something which is (covertly) contained in this concept A; or outside the concept A, although it does indeed stand in connection with it. In the one case I entitle the judgment analytic, in the other synthetic. Analytic judgments (affirmative) are therefore those in which the connection of the predicate with the subject is thought through identity; those in which this connection is thought without identity should be entitled synthetic... (sect. A7/B11, p. 48)[1]

Kant uses the example of the statement "All bodies are extended" (sect. A7/B11, p. 48) to demonstrate this point about subject and predicate relationships. For Kant, this statement represents an analytic judgment because it is not necessary to go beyond the notion of "extension" to see that "body" entails that idea. Bodies are by definition extended so it is reasonable to say that "extension" is in "body." In contrast, the statement "All bodies are heavy" is a synthetic judgment because "heavy" is not inherent in "body." As this example shows, analytic judgments are *a priori* in that no act of sensation will show that it is true; it is true prior to any experience:

---

[1]The *Critique of Pure Reason* was produced in two editions. In preparing the translation, Smith followed a convention whereby some passages from the first edition were retained and are labeled in the text with the letter A. Passages from the second edition are labeled with the letter B. For ease in locating passages across various editions, both the passage designation and page numbers from the Kemp-Smith version of the text are provided for references in this chapter.

> That a body is extended is a proposition that holds *a priori* and is not empirical. For, before appealing to experience, I have already in the concept of body all the conditions required for my judgment. I have only to extract from it, in accordance with the principle of contradiction,[1] the required predicate, and in so doing can at the same time become conscious of the necessity of the judgment—and that is what experience could never have taught me. On the other hand, though I do not include in the concept of a body in general the predicate 'weight', none the less this concept indicates an object of experience through one of its parts, and I can add to that part other parts of this same experience, as in this way belonging together with the concept. (Kant, 1965, B12, p. 49)

Kant introduces his primary problem concerning the need to substantiate the possibility of *a priori* synthetic statements and the distinction between analytic and synthetic statements, his subject-predicate form of this argument.

Transcendental Doctrine of the Elements

Kant proceeds to clarify the cognitive powers of the mind to uncover the means by which such judgments are possible. He looks first at the *a priori* elements involved in sensory knowledge. Kant's (1781/1965) *Critique of Pure Reason* is divided into two main parts: the Transcendental Doctrine of the Elements and the Transcendental Doctrine of Method. This chapter's focus will be primarily on the first section, which is further subdivided into the Transcendental Aesthetic and the Transcendental Logic. In the Transcendental Aesthetic, Kant introduces his idea of the pre-existing elements in the mind, that is, what he regards as the "science of all principles of *a priori* sensibility" (B36, p. 66). Kant proceeds to explore the principles of pure thought.

TRANSCENDENTAL AESTHETIC

Kant begins with the argument that the mind possesses the pre-existing intuitions of space and time. These primary intuitions are critical in the process of knowledge as they make sensation possible. In other words, space and time are not empirical elements; they cannot be observed or experienced directly in any way. Kant indicates that this view alone make geometry possible (space) as well as mathematics. Kant defines **intuition** as the means through which a mode of knowledge is in immediate relation to an object (p. 65), or as "that representation which can be given prior to all thought" (p. 153). This approach somewhat resembles that of Locke because it recognizes the power of the mind to quickly perceive an object presented to the mind. It is not the same as the "gut response" to which intuition refers in a colloquial sense or as often used by nurses. Instead it is a powerful cog-

---

[1] Here Kant refers to the philosopher Leibniz and his principle of contradiction (footnote not in original passage).

nitive process by which the mind reaches conclusions about its perceptions without there necessarily being a conscious cognitive problem-solving process in the situation. According to Kant, **space** and **time** are pure intuitions because they exist apart from experience. These *a priori* intuitions make experience possible.

This idea of space and time being prior to experience immediately is sure to cause some puzzled responses. Surely we can look at some objects with our three dimensional vision and see that one object is next to the other, or on top of the other; or one is nearer or farther away. That would seem to constitute an empirical recognition of what is referred to as space. According to Kant, this is not an appropriate realization, however, he considers such observations to support his position. Without some pre-existing idea of space, it would not be possible to ascertain relationships such as "next to" or "on top of" when exploring the relation of one object to another.

With this description, Kant presents a view where elements (appearances or phenomena) are furnished by objects and the intuitions of space and time remold these appearances into something suitable for thought. This does not constitute knowledge at this stage, however, because **knowledge** requires some way of pulling things together, what Kant refers to as Unity in consciousness. Without something to unify things in the mind, experiences become disjointed and knowledge does not become a part of the person united in one consciousness.

Hume (1748/1975, 1740/1978) argued that we cannot attribute anything more to experience than what we actually sense. For Kant, this would render knowledge impossible; there would be the rabble of the senses, as Plato commented, a chaotic "manifold" waiting to be ordered into some meaning. For Locke and Hume, the grouping of content is automatic because sensations spontaneously fall into some order. Kant disagrees arguing that the mind orders experience.

This focus on the mind as bringing order to experience presents a revolutionary idea in epistemology centered on the idea of a knowing subject. Experience must be experience for someone; "I think," therefore, is the ultimate condition of experience. Rather than being a passive recipient of sensory input, the mind takes an active role in constructing knowledge. This raises the possibility, however, that knowledge could be **subjective** in nature, individualized according to the thoughts and perspective of each unique person.

TRANSCENDENTAL LOGIC

Kant, however, does not see the potential for subjectivity as a problem. Although any experience must be an experience for someone, the mind does not act arbitrarily as it organizes experience. Instead this process is governed by principles in the mind. In the section of his work titled *Transcendental Logic*, Kant provides an inventory of these principles and how they make **objective** knowledge possible.

Once an experience or imagination is contained in thought, that is, perceived through the intuitions of Space and Time, categories that exist in the mind work to organize this input. Kant identified these categories, which he considers to be "pure concepts," as Quantity, Quality, Relation, and Modality. Although Aristotle considered such concepts to be derived from experience, for Kant these are *a priori* elements; they have no meaning of their own. They exist prior to experience and are present in the mind to be applied to experience; they provide an important mechanism by which experience can be created.

Because the categories exist in the mind prior to experience, it is possible to make *a priori* synthetic judgments. These categories enable knowledge of things beyond immediate consciousness. This process of making synthetic judgments involving things not immediately present to the person would not be possible if the mind operated only with empirical concepts and sensory experience.

Kant presents a view of knowledge that focuses on the processes of the mind as shown in Figure 5-1. In the knowing subject (the human mind), the capacities of human thought interact with the pre-existing categories of the mind to produce the "synthetic unity" essential for knowledge. Through human thought, experiences of **sensibility** (either actual experience or imagination) are taken in with the intuitions of space and time; once the thought is constructed, the pre-existing categories structure that input according to the roles of the categories and synthesize the information into a unified whole that meets the rigorous criteria of "knowledge:

> All knowledge demands a concept, though that concept may, indeed, be quite imperfect or obscure. But a concept is always, as regards its form, something universal which serves as a rule. (Kant, 1781/1965, A106, p. 135)

Because the mind operates consistent with the categories, or rules, this knowledge is *not* subjective but meets the criteria of necessity expected to count as *knowledge*. According to Kant, "**categories** are **concepts** which prescribe laws *a priori* to appearances, and therefore to nature, the sum of all appearances" (B 163, p. 172). As rules and as they exist the same in every mind, knowledge obtained through this process has some truth value. Kant explains his view in detail, drawing a comparison between different approaches to truth including the relationship between knowledge, objects, and a logical approach to truth:

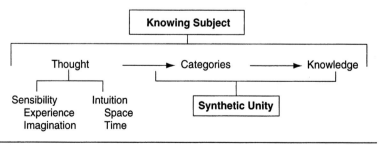

FIGURE 5-1. ◆ Basic elements of Kant's view of knowledge.

But, on the other hand, as regards knowledge in respect of its mere form (leaving aside all content), it is evident that logic, in so far as it expounds the universal and necessary rules of the understanding, must in these rules furnish criteria of truth. Whatever contradicts these rules is false. For the understanding would thereby be made to contradict its own general rules of thought, and so to contradict itself. These criteria, however, concern only the form of truth, that is, of thought in general; and in so far they are quite correct, but are not by themselves sufficient. For although our knowledge may be in complete accordance with logical demands, that is, may not contradict itself, it is still possible that it may be in contradiction with its object. The purely logical criterion of truth, namely, the agreement of knowledge with the general and formal laws of the understanding and reason, is a *condition sine qua non*, and is therefore the negative condition of all truth. But further than this logic cannot go. It has no touchstone for the discovery of such error as concerns not the form but the content. (Kant, 1781/1965, A60/B84, p. 98)

New Realm of Knowledge

Kant has proposed a fundamental shift in philosophy of knowledge (**epistemology**): the mind makes experience possible but experience is not the source of all knowledge. In spite of the mind's active role, the resulting knowledge is both necessary and universal, two conditions essential to refer to some bit of information as "knowledge." Moreover, such knowledge is possible without reliance upon sensory experience. This simplistic summary in no way reflects the complete contribution of Kant to philosophical thinking. It is important to remember that this line of thought, which addresses the possibility of knowledge beyond the limits of sensory experience, opened a vast new realm of possibilities for knowledge.

In spite of the new opportunities presented by this view, there are limits to the type of knowledge developed this way. Kant identifies two distinct realms of reality using the terms *phenomena* and *noumena*. The synthetic, *a priori* knowledge generated using the scheme described in the *Critique of Pure Reason* is knowledge only of the *phenomena*. Phenomena are *appearances*, or objects or aspects of reality as we experience them. This realm is quite distinct from the realm of *noumena*, or the things themselves, which are the actual objects in reality. According to Kant, knowledge is possible only for things as we experience them, the *phenomena*:

if we entitle certain objects, as appearances, sensible entities (phenomena), then since we thus distinguish the mode in which we intuit them from the nature that belongs to them in themselves, Now we must bear in mind that the concept of appearances, as limited by the Transcendental Aesthetic, already of itself establishes the objective reality of *noumena* and justifies the division of objects into *phaenomena* and *noumena*, and so of the world into a world of the senses and a world of the understanding (*mundus sensibilis et intelligibilis*), and

> indeed in such manner that the distinction does not refer merely to the logical form of our knowledge of one and the same thing, according as it is indistinct or distinct, but to the difference in the manner in which the two worlds can be first given to our knowledge, and in conformity with this difference, to the manner in which they are in themselves generically distinct from one another. For if the senses represent to us something merely *as it appears*, this something must also in itself be a thing, and an object of a non-sensible intuition, that is, of the understanding. (Kant, 1781/1965, pp. 266–267)

This complex description is presented succinctly in the *Prolegomena*, where Kant (1783/1902) points out that "the senses never and in no manner enable us to know things in themselves, but only their appearances, which are mere representations of the sensibility..." (p. 43).

Kant's ideology exceeds the boundaries of traditional **idealism**, which holds in simple form that there are no external objects, only our ideas of reality. In contrast, for Kant there certainly is an external reality with real objects that exist outside of the thinking subject. Knowledge of these objects, however, is limited to our perception of them, or the objects as they appear to us (*phenomena*). Kant (1783/1902) describes this distinction in the *Prolegomena*; he points out that the process of cognition that is the focus of his analysis:

> by no means excludes things of that sort (*noumena*), but rather limits the principles of the aesthetic (the science of the sensibility) to this, that they shall not extend to all things, as everything would then be turned into mere appearance, but that they shall only hold good of objects of possible experience. (p. 75)

Kant thus confirms that an external reality exists, but in the way humans view it, as it appears in space and time, it is *phenomenal* rather than concrete. Although the mind takes in reality in this manner, "the world, as appearance, though purely phenomenal, is not an arbitrary illusion, but governed by laws which render it necessary in all its details" (Carus, 1902, p. 199).

Implications

Kant's *Critique of Pure Reason*, one of the most challenging works in philosophy, is yet one of the most important that has been presented in Western writings. Kant produced numerous significant writings; his moral philosophy, in which he introduced what is referred to as the idea of the "categorical imperative,"[1] is a landmark in the study of ethics. Discussion of his views on ethics and moral reasoning is

---

[1]Kant's categorical imperative generally holds as the "fundamental law of the pure practical reason" that one should "Act so that the maxim of thy will can always at the same time hold good as a principle of universal legislation." (*Critique of Practical Reason*, available widely).

beyond the focus in this chapter, where the concern is to provide a very brief overview of some ideas that Kant contributed to the development of western epistemology.

The magnitude, complexity, and significance of Kant's work cannot be discussed sufficiently in such a straightforward venue as this chapter. It is perhaps most appropriate to focus on the major ideas presented by Kant and his overall contributions. Later developments in philosophy may seem to have clearer application or practical utility. Yet much of what transpired following Kant's writings can be traced directly or indirectly to the writings of this remarkable philosopher. Even Kant (1781/1965) presented his ideas as analogous to a Copernican Revolution in philosophy especially in the realm of metaphysics (p. 25). Kant follows the idea of previous philosophers when he opens his text with the statement "there can be no doubt that all our knowledge begins with experience." He continues, noting that "it does not follow that it all arises out of experience" (B 1, p. 41). Sensory experience is an important component of knowledge. Unlike the empiricists, however, Kant sees a definite possibility for knowledge that does not originate in experience.

Undoubtedly this brief overview of some significant points in Kant's ideas about knowledge will prompt a great deal of confusion for readers. That may be an inherent and somewhat unavoidable outcome in dealing with this philosopher's work. The views presented in the *Critique of Pure Reason* are widely regarded as some of the most difficult in philosophy (Carus [1902] refers to part of it as "unintelligible," p. 202). Kant uses awkward terminology and applies it in unique ways. He also wrote primarily for an academic audience. He was a philosopher by education and career and likely did not intend for nonacademics to comprehend his writings. The difficulty of his work is compounded by the need for translation and the fact that many words do not have exact translations across languages.

Phenomenology

In spite of these barriers, Kant's writing had a significant impact on later philosophical developments. One area of continuing emphasis that has been significant in many contexts, including nursing and other fields using qualitative research techniques, is in the development of the philosophy known as phenomenology. Phenomenology exists in a number of various forms, beginning with the writings of Hegel and Husserl among others and later adopted by the existentialist philosophers such as Heidegger and Merleau-Ponty. More recent philosophers and especially research methodologists have presented interesting blends of hermeneutics (see Chapter 10) and phenomenology, drawing from the works of more recent philosophers such as Gadamer (1975, 1976, 1981) and Ricouer (1974, 1981). A thorough discussion of the myriad nuances of phenomenology would constitute a life's work. It is a complex and in many respects convoluted combination of philosophy and methodology, and the subject matter has been covered very well in a number of introductory texts. For purposes of this discussion, it is most important to recognize some basic principles that underlie phenomenology in general along with the impact of this philosophical development on forms of inquiry in general.

In a broad sense, Phenomenology is derived from the idea of appearances, which is presented early in Greek philosophy in Plato's (1984) allegory of the Cave and further expounded by Kant. The philosophy of phenomenology emphasizes the interplay between objects and perception: aspects of reality are contributed by and thus shaped by the human experience and that experience is in turn shaped by the events or objects. In some of the literature of phenomenology, this interchange is referred to as the idea of "co-constitution," in that people and objects all are mutually constituted by the other. People shape their realities and these realities shape the people in return. Phenomenology is focused on "the things themselves," describing the totality of the "lived experience" of an individual in regard to some situation or occurrence. To the phenomenologist, there is little if any merit to studying learning, grief, heart attack, or childbirth as an *object* of experience; instead that object (or phenomenon) can only be understood by examining it as it is *lived*, complete with the elements contributed by the individual situation and context. The challenge for the phenomenological researcher is to understand the phenomenon in its entirety by sorting out what parts are contributed, what belong to the "thing itself" as part of its essential structure, and what other elements are derived from other aspects of experience. Grief, for example, could be objectified and studied as a concrete object. However, attempts to do so have been fraught with limitations. Such an approach not only reduces grief to components with numerical values or descriptors, it fails to recognize that grief is context-bound, that it does not occur outside of the experience of the one who is working through the grief. Grief as it is "lived" may be considerably different from grief captured on paper or in a laboratory type setting.

A phenomenological approach would explore the experience of grief as people live through or with it (the "lived experience"). Phenomenology, in general, is a search for the "essence" of the experience: in this example, grief and the basic structures that make it what it *is* (what makes it *grief*). The emphasis is on things as they first appear, before we attempt to know them as objects in "some impersonal or detached fashion" (Kearney, 1994, p. 13). Such an approach requires an elaborate, systematic, and comprehensive examination of the phenomenon, its essential components, and the aspects or elements contributed by the context or experience of the phenomenon.

Such an approach, which is focused on how an individual experiences a phenomenon, might initially seem quite subjective. In phenomenological inquiry, however, there is a desire to identify what is "objective" in studying the phenomenon. Ideas, values, beliefs, emotions, etc., cannot be allowed to intrude on or otherwise influence the processes or outcomes of inquiry. Phenomenological researchers typically engage in a process called "bracketing" to account for their own ideas about the subject of study. "Bracketing" has been interpreted by many researchers as the mere "setting aside" of preconceived ideas by the researcher. The process is sometimes mentioned in a rather dismissive manner by persons using other forms of qualitative research methods as a means to substantiate the credibility (that is, the nonsubjective nature) of the inquiry. This is troublesome for two reasons. One, it is questionable whether it is ever possible to completely set aside personal beliefs when engaged in inquiry. More important, however, phenomenological philosophy does not support such an idea. According to Husserl (1970), bracketing is the first step of phenomenological *reduction*. To view the phenomenon as it appears, the phenomenologist must identify all existing ideas that are overlaid on the phenomenon without the added layers of prejudices and subjective interpretations. Nurses have used variations of phenomenological research to study phenomena as diverse as caring for a chronically ill child (Gravelle, 1997), the work of clinical nurse consultants (Walters, 1996), and the nature of the discipline and practice of nursing (Paley, 1997).

 ## CONCLUSION

Kant provided a critical foundation for the development of philosophy and methodology based on his discussion of *phenomena* and *noumena* and the idea that objects of experience take on unique elements through the experience of them or through how they appear. This thesis provides a foundation as well for the development of the social sciences often referred to in philosophy as the *Geisteswissenschaften*, a German term used to refer broadly to knowledge of humans, in contrast to *Naturwissenschaften*, or the natural sciences. Husserl saw phenomenology as a strong call for rigor in all science despite what might seem to be a subjective component in this philosophy. According to Husserl, the natural science model based on empiricism attempted to maintain an "objective" stance, yet this objectivism was quite naïve because it failed to take account of existing conceptions and biases (Husserl, 1964; Kearney, 1994).

In developing his philosophy of phenomenology during the late 1800s, Husserl saw this philosophy falling clearly within the realm of epistemology. His emphasis on "consciousness" provided a focus on knowledge and the processes by which knowledge can be gained because it is a "consciousness-of-the-world" (Husserl, 1970; Kearney, 1994, p. 30). Heidegger, a student of Husserl, interpreted this experience from the standpoint of *being* rather than of *consciousness*. That is, Heidegger focused on the experience of living, rather than on how things can be known. This development from the foundation provided by Husserl contributes to some variations on phenomenology that exist in both the philosophy and the research methodology. In nursing this work appears primarily in the use of Heideggerian Hermeneutic methods for inquiry (Diekelmann, 2001; Draucker & Madsen, 1999; Nelms, 1996; Walters, 1995).

Other philosophers contributed to the development of phenomenology in a number of ways; all give impetus for the exploration of human existence as it is lived complete with individual, contextual, and unique aspects of all situations.

Perhaps because of the similarities between phenomenology as a research method and other forms of social research (i.e., other qualitative research modes), the intricate and important philosophical roots of phenomenology are not always apparent in phenomenological research. Paley (1997) argued that nurse researchers have demonstrated a poor understanding of Husserl's concepts of phenomenological philosophy and, thus, misapply these concepts in research; Paley similarly questioned applications of Heideggerian phenomenology (Paley, 1998). Nonetheless, elements of phenomenology as a philosophy and as a research methodology are abundant in nursing. All including Kant give credence to the focus of inquiry in nursing involving a complex combination of empirical and nonempirical elements, objects as they appear in addition to how they are lived and the meanings they have. This philosophy can only open the door to further exploration of the possibilities of knowledge.

 FOR DISCUSSION

1. Describe the differences and similarities between synthetic and analytic knowledge in reference to these types of knowledge in nursing.
2. How might Kant's views of synthetic knowledge contribute to knowledge development in nursing?
3. Discuss Kant's idea of objectivity and how synthetic knowledge can be objective due to the categories that exist in the mind. Develop supporting argument for and against this position.

REFERENCES

Carus, P. (1902). Essay on Kant's philosophy. In *Prolegomena to any future metaphysics that can qualify as a science* (P. Carus, Trans., pp. 167–240). La Salle, IL: Open Court.

Diekelmann, N. (2001). Narrative pedagogy: Heideggerian hermeneutical analyses of lived experiences of students, teachers, and clinicians. *Advances in Nursing Science, 23*(3), 53–71.

Draucker, C. B., & Madsen, C. (1999). Women dwelling with violence. *Image: The Journal of Nursing Scholarship, 31*, 327–332.

Gadamer, H. (1975). *Truth and method* (G. B. A. J. Cumming, Trans.). New York: Seabury Press.

Gadamer, H. (1976). On the scope and function of hermeneutical reflection (G. B. Hess & R. E. Palmer, Trans.). In D. E. Linge (Ed.), *Philosophical hermeneutics* (pp. 18–43). Berkeley: University of California Press.

Gadamer, H. (1981). *Reason in the age of science*. Cambridge, MA: MIT Press.

Gravelle, A. M. (1997). Caring for a child with a progressive illness during the complex chronic phase: parent's experience of facing adversity. *Journal of Advanced Nursing, 25*, 738–745.

Hume, D. (1975). *An enquiry concerning human understanding and an enquiry concerning the principles of morals* (L. A. Selby-Bigge, Ed., 3rd rev. ed., P. H. Nidditch, Ed.). Oxford: Oxford University Press. (Original work published 1748).

Hume, D. (1978). *A treatise of human nature* (L. A. Selby-Bigge, Ed., 2nd rev. ed, P. Nidditch, Ed.). Oxford: Oxford University Press. (Original work published 1740).

Husserl, E. (1964). *The idea of phenomenology* (W. P. Alston & G. Nakhnikian, Trans.). The Hague: Nijhoff.

Husserl, E. (1970). *The crisis of European sciences and transcendental phenomenology: An introduction to phenomenological philosophy* (D. Carr, Trans.). Evanston, IL: Northwestern University Press.

Kant, I. (1965). *Critique of pure reason* (N. K. Smith, Trans.). New York St. Martin's Press. (Original work published 1781).

Kant, I. (1902). *Prolegomena to any future metaphysics that can qualify as a science.* (P. Carus, Trans.). La Salle, IL: Open Court Publishing Company. (Original work published 1789)

Kearney, R. (1994). *Modern movements in European philosophy* (2nd Ed.). Dover, NH: Manchester University Press.

Nelms, T. P. (1996). Living a caring presence in nursing: a Heideggerian hermeneutical. *Journal of Advanced Nursing, 24,* 368–374.

Paley, J. (1997). Husserl, phenomenology and nursing. *Journal of Advanced Nursing, 26,* 187–193.

Paley, J. (1998). Misinterpretive phenomenology: Heidegger, ontology and nursing research. *Journal of Advanced Nursing, 27,* 817–824.

Plato. (1984). *The dialogues of Plato* (R. E. Allen, Trans.). New Haven, CT: Yale University Press.

Ricoeur, P. (1974). *The conflict of interpretations: Essays in hermeneutics.* Evanston, IL: Northwestern University Press.

Ricoeur, P. (1981). *Hermeneutics and the human sciences.* Paris, France: Cambridge University Press.

Walters, A. J. (1995). A Heideggerian hermeneutic study of the practice of critical care nurses. *Journal of Advanced Nursing, 21,* 492–497.

Walters, A. J. (1996). Being a clinical nurse consultant: A hermeneutic phenomenological reflection. *International Journal of Nursing Practice, 2*(1), 2–10.

Modern Science: Mirror of Reality

The philosophical school known as Logical Positivism provided the basis for most scientific development during the 20th century. This chapter focuses on the significant transitions caused by the emergence of this new philosophy and its effects in more recent times. In taking major leaps through time, it would be quite shortsighted to think that nothing significant happened in the interim between Kant and the rise of Positivism. Philosophical thought is fluid and evolves continuously, influencing and being influenced by events taking place in the larger context. Rather than give the impression that nothing significant happened in this interval, attention here is directed to the next major movement that influenced the development of nursing; this tradition known as Logical Positivism is an alternative to exploring the more subtle events along the way.

THE DEVELOPMENT OF LOGICAL POSITIVISM

Before becoming immersed in this tradition, however, it is important to understand how Logical Positivism evolved. Philosophy, as with all human creations, occurs within a social context. It is both influenced by and in turn influences further developments. Awareness of this relationship is particularly important in understanding Logical Positivism and subsequent philosophies. With Logical Positivism, the significance of the context is related to the fact that this philosophy demarcated a clear realm of knowledge referred to as *science* from this time forward. Previously much philosophical discussion in this regard had been focused on knowledge in general along with some attention to cosmology and the origins and structure of the universe. Epistemology flourished and became a focus in philosophical discussions. In much of these early writings, the terms **science** and **knowledge** were used interchangeably.

With the arrival of the 20th century, however, new discoveries and developments promoted the emergence of science as a distinct entity. Philosophy, in turn, demonstrated its own shift to the philosophy of science as a distinct area of philosophy. The rapid progress in scientific advancement led to the development of a specific branch of philosophy to support the continuing growth of science. In fact, one purpose of this movement was to create a "unified science," applying principles of science to all domains including philosophy so that they too could be considered "science."

The development of Logical Positivism and the emergence of a distinct realm of philosophy known as Philosophy of Science followed a complex and evolutionary path. The work of Kant had provided to a great extent a sort of turning point in philosophy. Kant's distinction between *phenomena* (objects as they appear to or are experienced by humans) and *noumena* (the objects themselves) contributed to a corresponding bifurcation in philosophy. The phenomenal realm was consistent with the tradition of **Idealism**. This tradition holds basically that there is no external world; all that exists are ideas of the world. While Kant clearly eschewed strict Idealism, his discussion of phenomena and the limits of knowledge certainly furthered inquiry along the lines of phenomenology and Idealism. There were elements in Kant's philosophy, however, that contributed to the eventual development of Logical Positivism. Acknowledging that an external reality did exist, Kant also fueled the emergence of materialistic and empiricist philosophies in addition to adding impetus to further development of Idealism.

The incentive for continuing work in the area of empiricism only became stronger with the incredible accomplishments that occurred under the rubric of science following Kant's time. By the early 1900s, a sort of philosophical crisis had emerged. The "new physics," represented by quantum theory and the theory of relativity, presented a significant challenge to existing philosophy. Such advances were showing tremendous potential for improving understanding of the world as well as having an incredible impact on human life. Yet existing philosophical systems either were not supportive or, in some cases, were not compatible with the science of the times. This context of the new physics, emerging economic theory, the industrial revolution, and major technical advances in general (consider the impact of electricity on human life) made it clear that a new philosophy of science was needed to support continuing progress.

Comte's Positivism

Logical Positivism is the philosophy that came to dominate this new era. The term **"Positivism"** actually was used many years earlier by Auguste Comte. Comte (1848/1953) had presented a theory of human development, arguing that societies pass through three distinct stages: theological, metaphysical and, finally, the positive stage. As a social theory, Positivism described how people give credit to explanations about the world around them. In the theological stage, elements of existence are explained in regard to the existence of deities or supernatural forces. The metaphysical stage provides explanations through abstract entities such as energies or ideas. Finally in the positive stage, people come to understand that there are scientific principles that explain the workings of the world. Knowledge is gained through experimentation and testing of hypotheses.

According to Comte (1848/1953), "the great object which Positivism sets before us individually and socially, is the endeavor to become more perfect" (p. 6). Comte expected this philosophy to "find a welcome in those classes only whose good sense has been left unimpaired by our vicious system of education, and whose generous sympathies are allowed to develop themselves freely" (pp. 3–4). Women and members of the working classes were the least likely to be educated at that time and so were less subject to the "impairment" created by the educational system. As a result, members of these groups were thought to be the source of greatest support for this new ideology that blended philosophy and politics.

Incorporating Logic into Positivism

Comte's Positivism was altered by an additional emphasis on logic and mathematics in the new philosophy of Logical Positivism. This movement had its early roots in 1907 when mathematician Hans Hahn, economist Otto Neurath, and physicist Philipp Frank met as an informal group to discuss philosophy of science. Their discussion included a focus on how science might be constructed to give appropriate recognition to the roles of mathematics, logic, and theoretical physics in describing experience. The group became known as the **"Vienna Circle"** when Moritz Schlick was invited to occupy the position of Professor of Philosophy of the Inductive Sciences at the University of Vienna in 1922. According to Ayer (1959), who was intricately involved with some of the later work of the Vienna Circle, the members of this group initially comprised "more of a club than an organized movement" (p. 3). The group emerged primarily on the basis of a shared interest and a common intellectual approach to problems. As the members continued to meet and discuss their views, the informal activities were augmented "by other activities which transformed the club into something more nearly resembling a political party" (p. 4). The group produced publications that provided details of the members' views, worked jointly with members of another similar group called the Berlin Circle, and organized international meetings held on a regular basis throughout the 1930s. The Vienna Circle, as a formal group, ended its weekly meetings in 1932 following the death of Schlick (Ayer, 1959, p. 5). The group essentially dissolved after the mid-1930s but their work left an extremely influential and enduring legacy.

As noted previously, Positivism holds the highest regard for facts, empirical data, and experiments as the basis of science. The "Logical" Positivists included the term "logical" to reflect their intent to capitalize on advancements in symbolic logic developed by Frege, Russell, and others.[1] They developed a set of rules and a particular view of language to guide philosophical development. The Logical Positivists placed an emphasis on *prescribing* how knowledge development *should* occur rather than on *describing* the processes of human cognition and knowledge. As noted previously, the intent was to promote the development of science and to raise all disciplines to a "scientific" level. The rules generated by these influential thinkers created a structure for the conduct of philosophy as well as for the advancement of knowledge.

 ## BASIC TENETS OF LOGICAL POSITIVISM

Rejection of Metaphysics

The Logical Positivists' primary concern was the reshaping of philosophy as a productive and meaningful activity. One of the first hurdles to be overcome in this mission involved the pitfalls of metaphysical concerns. The Logical Positivists believed that philosophers had focused for too long on discussion of absolutes, essences, transcendence, form, and other similar subject matter. The problem with such discussions was that statements made about ideas of this type could not be verified using logic or by collecting empirical data. For the Logical Positivists, however, a statement could be meaningful only if it could be verified in one of these ways. Statements had to be capable of being determined either True or False to be of any value. What, in fact, would be the purpose of saying anything if it were not possible to determine if the statement were true or not? Philosophy would

---

[1]Gottlob Frege and Bertrand Russell were noted philosophers whose significant contributions to the development of ideas about language and logic were beneficial to the analytic philosophy of the Logical Positivists.

need to rid itself of the trappings of metaphysics to function as a legitimate form of knowledge. The first tenet of Logical Positivism was the rejection of philosophical or metaphysical statements. According to this tradition, there simply was no purpose in pursuing such questions.

Role of Language

As a part of this idea about statements and verification, the Logical Positivists also generated a particular view of language. The relationship between elements of language and facts is important in determining if a statement makes sense or is capable of being verified by facts. The prominent 20th-century philosopher Ludwig Wittgenstein (1933/2001) had presented an elaborate view of language based on correspondence with facts and published in the *Tractatus Logico-Philosophicus*. This view was important in the Logical Positivists' formulation of their rules concerning language and the link between language and observation (Hempel, 1959). The resulting tenet is referred to as the idea of "**cognitive significance meaning,**" in other words, what Ayer (1959) refers to as "the famous slogan that the meaning of a proposition is its method of verification" (p. 13). This rule calls first of all for a proposition to be expressed in elementary or simple statements. Then the statement is evaluated with regard to the ability to verify the objects or empirical referents of the words in the statement. Such statements must be directly related to things that could be observed (empirical data).

This **verifiability principle,** as with many of the guiding tenets of Logical Positivism, was found to present too many difficulties and challenges. As a result, it later was replaced with an emphasis on the *possibility* of verification, in other words, that a statement needs only to be *capable* of being verified and not that it needs to be completely verified to be of any significance or value. This adoption of a slightly less stringent criterion may have been of small help, however, in the effort to develop knowledge because it still required a close relationship between words and facts.

Unification of Science

The Logical Positivists also presented their idea of a **unified science,** in other words, their belief that all science was to be viewed using the same principles. The Vienna Circle did not support distinctions among different classifications of science such as natural or social science; the same rules of science applied to all. Even ethics, if it were to be regarded as having any "scientific" base, would have to fit the mold of the other sciences. Philosophy as well was to be based on the "logic of science," particularly the analysis of language to determine what made it meaningful to state certain things (Carnap, 1956).

In summary the major tenets of Logical Positivism include the rejection of metaphysics, the importance of verifiability and language, and the idea of the possibility of a unified science. With these guiding principles, philosophy took on a prescriptive role, providing direction for what was thought to be increased progress in science. The philosophy continued to grow and change eventually creating a lasting influence on ideas concerning knowledge and especially theory development in all scientific disciplines

 # LOGICAL POSITIVISM AND THEORY DEVELOPMENT

Logical Positivism also led to a strong emphasis on theory development in science. The existence of verified theory actually was considered to be one hallmark of a science according to the Logical Positivists in that the knowledge of the science was organized into parsimonious and concise statements ideally showing law-like relationships among components. In general, development of a particular science was to proceed along a cumulative and linear path, articulating and expanding the theory, building on previous testing to improve the utility of the knowledge developed in explaining and predicting occurrences.

Theory and Language

One requirement that Logical Positivism imposed was that scientific theory first had to be based on **"first order language,"** using mathematics and symbolic logic to express the statements (propositions) of a theory. Statements of the theory also contained constants or terms that could be divided into two categories: observational or theoretical. Observational vocabulary represented entities that could be observed directly such as a physiologic measure or laboratory value. Theoretical vocabulary did not pertain to a specific observable entity or object. Such theoretical entities, however, needed to be interpreted in reference to observable, concrete things or events. Ultimately the truth value of a theory was determined using the principles of correspondence; the statements were true or not true based on how well they matched or corresponded with observable facts. This **correspondence theory of truth** provided the criterion for the verifiability need described earlier as it mandated the empirical testing of theories as the mode of verification during theory development.

Theory as a Tool of Prediction

Other considerations for science that are part of the Logical Positivist view of science are less obvious in this philosophy yet are clearly evident in the writings of philosophers associated with this tradition. The requirements for theory indicate an emphasis on theory as a tool for prediction. By developing axioms from descriptions, it would be possible not only to explain events but to predict them as well. This philosophy led to the common understanding that the purpose of science was to "predict, explain, and control" events. Indeed this is the basis of the view of experimental or quasi-experimental research as presented in many research methods texts in nursing as well as in other disciplines. The researcher develops an intervention, for example, an educational offering, an exercise program, or perhaps a new wound dressing procedure. A research design is developed that enables the researcher to determine what effects the intervention has on the subjects in the study. If conducted properly with appropriate sampling techniques and controls, the researcher can have considerable faith in the accuracy of the results. Through such research, investigators contribute an understanding of cause and effect relationships and can expect particular outcomes when they use the intervention in the future. Carrying this thinking a bit further, it is presumed possible to control outcomes in a sense by introducing certain "causes" or interventions to produce a desired result. According to Logical Positivism, this is the primary purpose of science: to predict, explain, and control occurrences.

Hypotheticodeductive Model

Hempel (1952) described this process of theory development and testing in great detail and presented a procedure widely referred to as the **hypotheticodeductive model** of research. The name of this procedure captures the basic elements of this form of science. The scientist deduces hypotheses from an existing "proven" theory and subjects these to appropriate research and testing. The results provide important information that is used to clarify the original theory and to identify the need for modification. Additional hypothesis testing would continue to shape the theory, generating a product of increased accuracy and breadth as the hypotheses were tested in new situations or with different phenomena. This process can be described as a cumulative, linear approach because knowledge proceeds along the same linear path in a cumulative manner presumably with incremental increases in theory development.

This emphasis shows a clear connection to the work of the 17th century empiricists. For the empiricists, the advancement of knowledge took place through the collection of facts and the proper ordering and examination of facts, as Bacon enthusiastically and eloquently advocated. Proper ordering comes from systematic experimentation and data analysis. For Logical Positivism to accomplish its aims, a key element of this process is the idea of the "**autonomy of facts**": facts must be capable of examination, collection, ordering, in isolation from their context. In other words, "facts" exist autonomously without any influence from their relationship with context or other facts. The collection of what might be called, in this sense, "pure" facts required also that scientists be completely "**value-free**" in their work. For this system of science to work properly, scientists were expected to work unfettered by any personal and supposedly theoretical bias.

The idea of viewing facts in isolation, as autonomous entities, is a form of **reduction**, a dominant feature in the "received view." Not only is the world reduced to the isolated units referred to as facts, knowledge of the world should be successively reduced to the most basic sciences and the most inclusive theories. Later theories subsume early theories; as science progresses, more simple statements come to include the earlier, more elaborate theories. The ultimate goal of this process was to produce simple, parsimonious statements of theory that included as many aspects of the world as possible (Hempel, 1952).

LOGICAL POSITIVISM'S INFLUENCE ON NURSING

Logical Positivism evolved over a nearly 40-year period and its history is embedded in countless essays, articles, and books. The movement's own members and staunchest supporters were responsible for the many changes over time.

The major tenets of Logical Positivism (Box 6-1) have had a strong influence on the development of science. Nursing science certainly was not able to avoid this influence. This occurred, in part, because many of the most influential nurse leaders were educated and socialized in disciplines steeped in its ideology. It also is the case, however, that Logical Positivism was so ubiquitous that it would have been difficult to avoid its grasp in any knowledge-building enterprise. Strengthening the influence of this ideology, there also can be no doubt that incredible achievements occurred consistent with at least part of this philosophical orientation.

Webster, Jacox, and Baldwin (1981) declared this philosophy "dead" in a book chapter published in 1981; in spite of stipulating the demise of the philosophy, they described the continuing influence of this view on nursing by referring to the lingering "ghost" of the philosophy. While Logical Positivism may have been supplanted by numerous subsequent evolutions of philosophical thought, there can be no question that its remnants influenced nursing knowledge development for some time.

This general philosophy of Logical Positivism and its later iterations typically are referred to as the **"received view"** (Suppe, 1977) of science. In nursing, the influence is evident particularly in the historical development of the discipline and

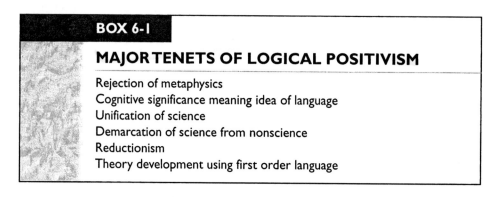

BOX 6-1

MAJOR TENETS OF LOGICAL POSITIVISM

Rejection of metaphysics
Cognitive significance meaning idea of language
Unification of science
Demarcation of science from nonscience
Reductionism
Theory development using first order language

BOX 6-2

INFLUENCE OF LOGICAL POSITIVISM

Correspondence theory of truth
Emphasis on empirical verification
Hypotheticodeductive model of science
Focus on theory and product of science rather than process
Context of discovery irrelevant
Autonomy of facts (facts can be viewed out of context)
Emphasis on objectivity and value-free nature of science

the theory development movement of the 1960s and 1970s. In the 1960s, advanced education for nurses, particularly at the doctoral level, was focused to a great extent on education in the basic sciences because few programs were available that led to a doctoral degree in nursing. Debate raged, however, over the relationship between nursing knowledge and knowledge in other disciplines, particularly the "basic sciences." During the late 1950s and early 1960s, the Division of Nursing Resources of the U.S. Public Health Service developed programs to provide financial support for nurses seeking academic advancement and research training (Kalisch & Kalisch, 1978). These programs enabled a large number of nurses to obtain doctoral degrees in disciplines presumably *related* to nursing, where they were socialized and educated in the philosophies and methods of those disciplines. It also, however, coincided with the peak of the influence of Logical Positivism in other sciences (Box 6-2).

Theory Development

In nursing, one easily seen result was a strong emphasis on theory development. Logical Positivism required that knowledge be organized into theories and that those theories have a particular structure and appearance. To obtain status as a science, nurses worked diligently to explore the origins of nursing knowledge and to develop theoretical formulations to guide further research and development of the discipline.

In the 1960s, the Division of Nursing, a branch of the U.S. Public Health Service, provided funding for conferences on theory development for nursing. Two such conferences were held; Case Western Reserve University sponsored the first in 1968 and the University of Colorado hosted the second in 1969. The proceedings from these conferences reveal the emphasis on delineating the nature of the discipline and science of nursing and the use of philosophy to provide direction for further development. As Silva and Rothbart (1984) pointed out, writings during this time showed the influence of Logical Empiricism (or Logical Positivism) on the development of nursing during the 1960s and 1970s.

If nursing was to be considered a "science," it was critical that research be theory-based because theory was the desired product of a science for the Logical Positivists. This emphasis generated a considerable amount of discussion in the literature about the relationship between theory and research (Benoliel, 1977; Dickoff, James, & Wiedenbach, 1968a. 1968b; Fawcett, 1978) as well as a large volume of literature on theory development and evaluation (Chinn & Jacobs, 1978, 1983; Hardy, 1974, 1978; Kim, 1983, 1987; Newman, 1972; Walker & Avant, 1983). This emphasis on theory development dominated nursing in the late 1960s through the 1970s. Not surprisingly, this time frame includes the development of the initial nursing theories such as the work of Orlando (1961), Rogers (1970), Roy (1970, 1971) and others. These theoretical developments showed an effort to be consistent with the views of theory presented in Logical Positivism. The writings on theory showed a formalized view with an emphasis on axioms and propositions and quantitative testing of hypotheses derived from theory. Concepts needed to be defined in operational terms, showing their means of empirical testing. Descriptive studies were of value but only to the extent they provided "baseline data" for subsequent theory building (Fawcett, 1978, p. 60).

Limitations of Logical Positivism in Nursing Theory Development

Webster, Jacox and Baldwin (1981) contend that "undue adherence to the positions and ideas of the Received view has stilted the development of nursing theories" (p. 34). Nursing's allegiance with disciplines heavily immersed in this narrow philosophy of science led to an over-reliance on its guidance for knowledge development. Similarly there seemed to be a lack of awareness of alternative views of science even as other disciplines were discussing broader views, particularly those of Kuhn (1962, 1970, see Chap. 7).

Because of major developments in philosophy and in nursing as a discipline, it might be reasonable to assume that Logical Positivism is no longer of any influence in nursing. While it fails to dominate discussions of nursing knowledge, the continuing legacy of the received view cannot be dismissed. Webster, Jacox, and Baldwin referred to the "ghost" of the received view more than 20 years ago, and some of that specter continues. As a result of Logical Positivism, a considerable vocabulary was developed in nursing and a wide base of dogma continues to appear in nursing conversations. Distinctions between art and science, references to boundaries around disciplines and the uniqueness of nursing, Truth as a goal of science and a requirement for objectivity are derived from this philosophy and are a continuing part of nursing knowledge development (Rodgers, 1991). Perhaps most important, however, the Logical Positivism movement provided major incentive for examination of the knowledge base of nursing and the development of nursing as a discipline.

Despite the movement's significance and Logical Positivism's strong influence on a number of disciplines, significant limitations ultimately led to its demise. The movement's major tenets were found to be plagued with weaknesses. In general, the requirement that knowledge be organized into rigidly formal theories that could be expressed using principles of logic and calculus proved to be a nearly impossible goal for many disciplines. Such a requirement also failed to place sufficient value on less organized or formal knowledge, which might be useful or meaningful in a discipline even without the formality of theory. The requirement of correspondence as the criterion for evaluating the truth of a theory presented problems as well. Scholars were compelled to develop ways to "measure" phenomena of interest to make them amenable to verification through the collection of empirical data. For entities such as dignity, hope, and perhaps even pain, there are no clear empirical correlates. Scientists would, therefore, have to construct empirical definitions (observational definitions) for phenomena of interest, possibly leaving out or ignoring important aspects of the situation not amenable to such observation. Coping would become "coping as measured by the total score on the instrument" rather than an individual's description of his or her psychological, social, and behavioral responses to manage a difficult life situation. Certainly the first definition seems more exact, constructing coping in view of a numerical score. Further, elaborate procedures exist to substantiate the accuracy and relevance of that score. Yet that number undoubtedly fails to reflect the complexity and the scope of the human experience, thus rendering, by itself, a limited view of the experience isolated from its context. Where psychosocial phenomena are concerned, removing these phenomena from the context clearly has significant limitations for understanding in nursing. The same can be said, however, of physiologic parameters, such as physiologic measures for diabetes, which provide only one part of the puzzle of understanding control of diabetes.

Another limitation of Logical Positivism stemmed from its promotion of a cumulative, linear approach to knowledge. This process of scientists working using established theories and incrementally refining and expanding this theoretical foundation had the potential to promote progress in science by converging effort on promising, previously tested theories that were showing likelihood of success. In addition, with scientists focused on a limited number of theories, effort would be concentrated on specific areas of interest rather than diffused across a variety of areas of inquiry.

This same approach, however, can have an equally strong negative effect on progress. Proceeding according to a cumulative pattern can institutionalize and magnify error just as it might magnify progress (Fleck, 1935). Equally significant is the observation that it places no value on and leaves little room for creativity and innovation. There may be creativity within the prevailing focus of inquiry but support for pursuing paths and ideas beyond the existing norm is minimal if not completely absent. This is particularly troublesome in view of the fact that some highly significant scientific advances resulted either by accident or a scientist persevering in spite of direct opposition from a majority of the scientific community.

One striking example of science's reluctance to accept findings outside the realm of current emphasis is found in the work of Australian physicians Robin

Warren and Barry Marshall who were the first to identify *Helicobacter pylori* as a causative agent for ulcers in 1982. Eight years passed with the medical community resisting their findings before the National Institutes of Health (1994) presented a Consensus Development Conference and concluded there was, indeed, a strong connection between *H. pylori* and ulcers. Following that pronouncement, recommended treatment of peptic ulcer disease was revised to include the administration of antibiotics specific for *H. pylori*. Although antibiotics had been found previously to heal and prevent recurrence of the vast majority of ulcers, Warren and Marshall were compelled to experiment on themselves; they infected themselves with H. pylori and subsequently developed ulcers to garner the close attention of medical researchers. (On a more humorous note, Post-its® also were a bit of an accidental discovery. While not within the domain of more typical academic sciences, this development has had a tremendous impact on how people communicate and use bookmarks [Legacy of Innovation, 1998].) Both examples show the limitations of following a traditional, cumulative approach to knowledge development and the importance of innovative and accidental discoveries in promoting progress.

 ## CONCLUSION

It may seem, however, that the methods prescribed by Logical Positivism persist even to the present. It is important to recognize that the limitations of Logical Positivism are not necessarily a part of all research in which statistical analysis and hypothesis testing are employed. It is quite possible for a researcher to conduct research using a hypotheticodeductive model without believing that the results constitute Absolute Truth and without subscribing to the other tenets of Logical Positivism. Scientists also conduct research in ways that challenge prevailing wisdom although there often are barriers to doing so. Rigid adherence to the received view tends to be more a constructed view of science than a reality for scientists. While Logical Positivism as a philosophy was fraught with problems and unrealistic expectations, it did begin to define the unique role of science and provided an impetus for establishing scientific rigor and integrity.

In many disciplines, Logical Positivism began to fade as the dominant philosophy of science by the 1950s. This philosophy was determined even by some of its own supporters to be impossible to achieve and inconsistent with existing modes of progress in science. Logical Positivism attempted to prescribe how science *should* be conducted to maximize progress. An alternate view, however, was that science did operate and progress quite well and the proper role for philosophy was to *describe* rather than *prescribe* how it functioned. The emphasis subsequently shifted to understanding science rather than dictating its procedures.

FOR DISCUSSION

1. Compare and contrast the procedures of science advocated by the Logical Positivists with the "typical" research process followed by scientists.
2. Describe the goal(s) of science according to the Logical Positivists.
3. Identify the Logical Positivists' position on the nature of truth/Truth.
4. Discuss strengths and limitations of this approach to science.
5. Identify implications of this view for the development of the discipline of nursing. Consider different possibilities for the nature of the discipline of nursing in responding.

REFERENCES

Ayer, A. J., Ed. (1959). *Logical Positivism*. Glencoe, IL: Free Press.

Benoliel, J. Q. (1977). The interaction between theory and research. *Nursing Outlook, 25*, 108–113.

Carnap, R. (1956). *Meaning and necessity*. Chicago: University of Chicago Press.

Chinn, P. L., & Jacobs, M. K. (1978). A model for theory development in nursing. *Advances in Nursing Science, 1*(1), 1–11.

Chinn, P. L., & Jacobs, M. K. (1983). *Theory and nursing: A systematic approach*. St. Louis: Mosby.

Comte, A. (1953). *A general view of Positivism* (J. H. Bridges, Trans). Stanford, CA: Academic Reprints. (Original work published 1848).

Dickoff, J., & James, P., & Wiedenbach, E. (1968a). Theory in a practice discipline: Part I, practice-oriented theory. *Nursing Research 17*, 415–435.

Dickoff, J., & James, P., & Wiedenbach, E. (1968b). Theory in a practice discipline: Part II, practice-oriented theory. *Nursing Research 17*, 545–554.

Fawcett, J. (1978). The relationship between theory and research: A double helix. *Advances in Nursing Science, 1*(1), 49–62.

Fleck, L., Ed. (1935). *Genesis and development of a scientific fact*. Chicago: University of Chicago Press.

Hardy, M. E. (1974). Theories: Components, development, evaluation. *Nursing Research, 23*, 100–107.

Hardy, M. E. (1978). Perspectives on nursing theory. *Advances in Nursing Science, 1*(1), 27–48.

Hempel, C. G. (1952). *Fundamentals of concept formation in empirical science*. Chicago: University of Chicago Press.

Hempel, C. G. (1959). The empiricist criterion of meaning. In A. J. Ayer (Ed.), *Logical Positivism* (pp. 108–129). Glencoe, IL, Free Press.

Kalisch, P. A., & Kalisch, B. J. (1978). *The advance of American nursing*. Boston: Little, Brown.

Kim, H. S. (1983). *The nature of theoretical thinking in nursing*. Norwalk, CT: Appleton-Century-Crofts.

Kim, H. S. (1987). Structuring the nursing knowledge system: A typology of four domains. *Scholarly Inquiry for Nursing Practice, 1*, 111–114.

Kuhn, T. S. (1962). *The structure of scientific revolutions*. Chicago: University of Chicago Press.

Kuhn, T. S. (1970). *The structure of scientific revolutions* (2nd Ed.). Chicago: University of Chicago Press.

Legacy of Innovation. (1998). Art Fry and the invention of Post-it® Notes. *3M Innovation Chronicles*, April 1998 (available online http://www.3m.com/about3M/pioneers/fry.html) (Accessed March 4, 2004).

National Institutes of Health. (1994). *Consensus statement: Helicobacter pylori in peptic ulcer disease, 12*(1), February, 7–9.

Newman, M. A. (1972). Nursing's theoretical evolution. *Nursing Outlook, 20,* 449–453.

Orlando, I. (1961). *The dynamic nurse-patient relationship.* New York: G. P. Putnam's Sons.

Rodgers, B. L. (1991). Deconstructing the dogma in nursing knowledge and practice. *Image: The Journal of Nursing Scholarship, 23,* 177–181.

Rogers, M. E. (1970). *An introduction to the theoretical basis of nursing.* Philadelphia: F. A. Davis.

Roy, C. (1970). Adaptation: A conceptual framework for nursing. *Nursing Outlook, 18*(3), 42–45.

Roy, C. (1971). Adaptation: A basis for nursing practice. *Nursing Outlook 19,* 254–257.

Silva, M. C., & Rothbart, D. (1984). An analysis of changing trends in philosophies of science on nursing theory development and testing. *Advances in Nursing Science, 6*(2), 1–13.

Suppe, F. (1977). Historical background to the received view. In F. Suppe (Ed.), *The structure of scientific theories* (pp. 6–15). Urbana, IL: University of Illinois Press.

Walker, L. O., & Avant, K. C. (1983). *Strategies for theory construction in nursing.* Norwalk, CT: Appleton-Century-Crofts.

Webster, G., Jacox, A., & Baldwin, B. (1981). Nursing theory and the ghost of the received view. In J. C. McCloskey and H. K. Grace (Eds.), *Current issues in nursing* (pp. 26–35). Boston: Blackwell Scientific.

Wittgenstein, L. (2001). *Tractatus Logico-philosophicus.* (D. F. Pears and B. F. McGuinness, Trans.). London: Routledge. (Original work published 1933).

CHAPTER 7

Science in Context: Historicist Conceptualizations of Science

KEY IDEAS

absolutism	progress
anomalies	psychologism
conceptual problems	puzzle solving
crisis	relativism
incommensurable	research traditions
normal science	revolution
objectivism	science as process
paradigm	science as product
problem solving	weighting of problems

Following the gradual demise of Logical Positivism, Historicism was the next major tradition that gained prominence in Western philosophy of science. Historicism actually has a long history in philosophy although it did not develop a strong following in its earlier stages. The first significant use appears to be around the mid-1800s with more widespread use occurring after World War I.

OVERVIEW OF HISTORICISM

Many different views fall under the heading of Historicism. In general the tradition of Historicism is characterized by the belief that an adequate understanding of the nature and value of anything requires consideration of its place and role within a process of historical development. Historicism, therefore, provides both a methodological principle regarding how to understand situations as well as a philosophy about how situations came to exist. Historicism presents the view that understanding an event or situation requires that it be seen as part of a larger process. The key feature of Historicism in regard to philosophy of science is identical in that scientific developments must be examined in regard to the context in which they occurred (for example, the time, situation, and people involved). In keeping with this idea that context and history are important in evaluating knowledge claims, Historicists view science from a process standpoint. For Logical Positivists, science was evaluated on the basis of its product, particularly the theories developed through research. Historicists, in contrast, look at the process as a way to understand and evaluate science.

Historicism bears some similarity to a general philosophical position known as **Relativism**. As an epistemological position, Relativism holds that all knowledge claims must be evaluated *relative* to something. Typically claims are evaluated in regard to (or relative to) the context in which the claim was produced or the particular perspective of the individual or group making the claim. In the case of Historicism, Relativism enters into the evaluation of claims about science and truth to the extent that these claims need to be considered in view of the contexts and the perspectives from which the science emerged.

Relativist and historicist positions present a stark contrast to other philosophical views known as **Absolutism** and **Objectivism**. The term "absolutist" view is used primarily in regard to ethics and is the position that certain actions or behaviors are absolutely (i.e., always) wrong or always must be performed. In epistemology, the term Objectivism captures a similar idea. An objectivist view purports that knowledge claims are relevant to the objects about which a statement is made, not to the person(s) making the statement. In other words, Objectivism supports the possibility of knowledge claims without regard for the values or perspective of any individual person or group.

In an Absolutist position, there is only one definitive course of action; an objective position holds that it is possible to examine situations without bias or preconception and that there is some foundation for comparison of claims (that is, an objective reality that makes it possible to determine what is True). A relativist, in contrast, sees things more contextually or situationally. In nursing science, this distinction is most evident in regard to views of truth and the distinction between an absolute, necessary Truth, and truths that are more individualized. One negative connotation of such a relativistic view equates it with **psychologism**, rendering views as based merely on individual psychological prop-

---

BOX 7-1

HISTORICISM

Historicism, in regard to philosophy of science, places importance on the context and processes in which scientific activity takes place. Claims of truth, knowledge, or progress must be evaluated in regard to the context in which they were developed.

---

erties. Rather than reflect any actual knowledge, an extreme relativist position might be considered to reflect only an individual's unique position or opinion. A less radical view allows that perceptions and decisions sometimes require consideration of individual contexts and nuances (Box 7-1).

INFLUENCE OF THOMAS KUHN

Thomas Kuhn was in an ideal situation to consider the roles of history and context in the progression of science. Kuhn pursued graduate education in theoretical physics and spent 3 years as a Junior Fellow of the Society of Fellows of Harvard University (Kuhn, 1970, p. v). During that time he had the opportunity to study the history of science and read extensively in philosophy and psychology as well as a variety of scientific works in his own field.[1] This background may have afforded Kuhn unique credibility in regard to his work on philosophy of science. He was not a philosopher who had chosen to study the processes and contexts of science. Quite the contrary, he was a scientist, an insider so to speak, and stood in a rather privileged position to examine the workings of science. In addition, his field of theoretical physics held particular intrigue as an exemplary model of what might be called "real" or "hard" science. Kuhn, thus, had the perfect opportunity to examine the development of science and the context in which that scientific activity occurred.

Paradigms

Kuhn viewed science not as a theory development activity necessarily but as a process of **puzzle solving**. This puzzle solving activity occurs consistent with "**para-**

---

[1]One of the works that Kuhn describes as influential during this time is Ludwik Fleck's *Genesis and development of a scientific fact*. Fleck describes the development of the facts associated with syphilis, giving vivid insight into how things identified as fact actually carry with them lengthy conceptual and social histories.

digms" that guide scientists in determining how to proceed with their scientific activities. Kuhn presented countless definitions of paradigms in his work but subsequently clarified his use of the term to mean a "disciplinary matrix" along with "exemplars" relevant to that matrix. The disciplinary matrix is comprised of the shared elements of knowledge including beliefs, values, and substantive content (symbolic generalizations). The paradigm also includes exemplars, the concrete problem solutions that have been accepted by a scientific community. Exemplars pose a question and provide an indication of how the question might be answered. The sharing of the disciplinary matrix and exemplars (in other words, the paradigm) creates a community of scientists. Scientists agree on what problems are relevant as well as what counts as a solution.

The existence of a paradigm, according to Kuhn (1970), marks the maturity of a science:

> ...it is sometimes just its reception of a paradigm that transforms a group previously interested merely in the study of nature into a profession or, at least, a discipline. In the sciences (though not in fields like medicine, technology, and law, of which the principle *raison d'etre* is an external social need) the formation of specialized journals, the foundation of specialists' societies and the claim for a special place in the curriculum have usually been associated with a group's first reception of a single paradigm. (p. 19)[1]

When an established paradigm is present to guide continuing scientific activity, scientists are working in a manner referred to by Kuhn (1970) as "normal science." **Normal science** is the highly cumulative process of puzzle solving in which the paradigm guides scientific activity and the paradigm is, in turn, articulated and expanded. Research conducted as part of normal science "is directed to the articulation of those phenomena and theories that the paradigm supplies" (p. 24). A paradigm, particularly early in its acceptance, is not a successful answer to problems facing the discipline. Rather it is "at the start largely a promise of success..." (p. 25). Normal science, therefore, is the characteristic activity of scientists as they work to improve the paradigm under which they operate. This work of paradigm articulation involves a combination of experimental and theoretical activity.

In the absence of a paradigm, scientific activity exists in what Kuhn calls the preparadigm phase. In this phase, there is considerable debate over what problems to address, what methods are appropriate, and what standards should be applied to determine the effectiveness of proposed solutions to scientific problems. Scientific activity during this phase demonstrates confusion and lack of focus. Without a paradigm, all facts are "likely to seem equally relevant" because

---

[1]Kuhn makes a clear distinction between such "disciplines" or sciences as law and medicine, which exist to meet a specific need of societies, and the more traditional academic disciplines in regard to their emergence as fields of study. This distinction appears to have been overlooked in subsequent discussions of Kuhn's work in nursing.

there is no paradigm to govern identification and selection of facts to be gathered in inquiry. Early fact gathering, therefore, is "a far more random activity" and a great diversity of viewpoints pull the activity in different directions (p. 15).

ANOMALIES AND REVOLUTIONS

According to Kuhn, the paradigm is essential to provide direction and focus for activities. It is necessary also to enable interpretation of findings in the course of scientific activity. Not only does the paradigm provide a framework for making sense of results, it also enables scientists to determine if results are out of line with expectations. Kuhn refers to phenomena that are not accounted for by the paradigm as anomalies. Anomalies must be explained within the context of the paradigm because the paradigm must account for all relevant phenomena and content. The identification of anomalies then can be a great stimulus for inquiry and can focus scientific effort on their explanation.

The normal process of science may fail to account for or solve these anomalies so they can accumulate over time. When they become sufficient in number or importance, scientists confront a **crisis**. Normal science breaks down and the only way to account for anomalies will be to generate a new paradigm (Kuhn, 1970, pp. 74–75). A period of change occurs in which the anomalies are assimilated into existing scientific knowledge with a new paradigm generated to provide a coherent focus for subsequent scientific work. Scientists do not merely abandon a paradigm because anomalies exist; because of the critical role of the paradigm in science, it is essential that a new paradigm be created and supported to guide scientific activity. Scientists will declare the existing paradigm invalid only if a suitable alternative is available (p. 77).

Kuhn described the process of change from one paradigm to the replacement paradigm as a **revolution**. Anomalies create a crisis in science and a situation that resembles the preparadigm stage of the science. The revolution phase of science consists of a noncumulative episode in which the older paradigm is replaced in whole or in part by an incompatible new one. The change in paradigm also changes what scientists look at and what is seen; the world does not change but what the scientist sees in it does change. In that respect, the change in paradigm is much like a change in "world view."

This process, as described by Kuhn (1970), resembles the cumulative and linear nature of science advocated by the Logical Positivists. Scientists work within the boundaries of established paradigms to refine and expand the paradigm. This mechanism is similar to the Logical Positivists' process of expanding and refining a theory. Several significant differences are present that set Kuhn's ideas as very distinct from those of the Received View. One obvious difference exists in Kuhn's focus on paradigms rather than theories. Paradigms are considerably broader and include more components than theories alone. They may include theories but generally include elements that influence how the scientists view their world and the phenomena of interest to them.

The basis for change in paradigms is one of the most striking features of Kuhn's philosophy. In Logical Positivism, changes in theory occur as the result of repeated testing of hypotheses and the accumulation of facts to make appropriate refinement in the theory. For Kuhn, however, the process of paradigm change is not based on fact and there are no rules for deciding that one paradigm is necessarily better than another is. This is an unavoidable position, however, as paradigms are **incommensurable**, that is, scientists cannot directly compare one paradigm to another because each paradigm involves its own reality or its own view of the world. There is no independent factor, according to Kuhn, no objective foundation (such as Truth) that can be used to determine if one paradigm is "better" than another. In the absence of such decision rules or criteria, the decision to replace one paradigm with another is an act of judgment.

Kuhn points out that the process of choosing among paradigms "regularly raises questions that cannot be resolved by the criteria of normal science" (Kuhn, 1970, p. 109). This choice involves a question of values, particularly "which problems is it more significant to have solved?" (p. 110). Answering this question requires an appeal to criteria other than those typically associated with decision making in science.

PROGRESS IN SCIENCE

Progress is considered by some philosophers to be a critical feature of science. Scientific activity generally can be considered as continual movement toward something; truth, practicality, and usefulness provide a few examples. Kuhn (1970) reflects this belief as well in his statement that "to a very great extent the term 'science' is reserved for fields that do progress in obvious ways. Nowhere does this show more clearly than in the recurrent debates about whether one or another of the contemporary social sciences is really a science" (p. 160). Challenging the utility of such a "definition of 'science," he adds:

> Probably questions like the following are really being asked: Why does my field fail to move ahead in the way that, say physics does? What changes in techniques or method or ideology would enable it to do so? These are not, however, questions that could respond to an agreement on definition. (p. 160)

Returning to the question of progress, Kuhn concludes that in any community "the result of successful creative work *is* progress. How could it possibly be anything else?" (p. 160).

Kuhn's Contributions to Science and Nursing

It is reasonable to say that Kuhn, with his idea of scientific revolutions and paradigm changes, had the potential to revolutionize views of science. Other philosophers presented important views of science in the interim between Logical Positivism and Historicism.[1] Kuhn's (1970) view, however, provided a radical departure from these positions and opened an entire new realm for discussion of science.

SCIENCE AS A HUMAN ENTERPRISE

Prior views failed to capture contextual elements that are a major aspect of Kuhn's work. Particularly obvious in this regard is the human element. Progress in science, according to Kuhn, is not a matter of getting closer to Truth, collecting more empirical data, or creating "better" theories. Because assessment of such achievements is so highly dependent on individual determinations, progress is a matter of judgment.

This would seem to provide a picture of science as a highly subjective activity. Perhaps an accurate statement is that any activity involving humans and their decisions must have some element of subjectivity. Criteria that may have seemed objective, such as truth and falsehood, actually do involve the scientists' judgments to a great extent. According to Kuhn, the collection of facts that determine Truth claims is guided by preconceptions, either existing theory or the paradigm for Kuhn. The belief in objectivity, or what is commonly referred to as "value-free" science, is misguided. The defensible decision making of the members of the scientific community consequently becomes a focus in determining appropriate action and progress in the field.

Kuhn's view of science, organized around paradigm-driven normal science and subsequent scientific revolutions, presents science as a human enterprise bound by context and with scientists functioning as a community (see Box 7-2). Although the current notion of "community of scholars" generally has a slightly different slant such as the development of collaborative academic environments, it is easy to see how such an idea of community in nursing could contribute toward the development of nursing *science*. There is a clear resemblance to Kuhn's work in the idea of people working cooperatively toward shared goals and ideals. Because of variations in the outcomes of scientific activity, however, it is most appropriate to think of science in regard to its **process** rather than its **product**. In Kuhn's philosophy, the described process includes elements of the cumulative, linear approach presented by the Logical Positivists. One important element missing from a strictly Logical Positivist approach, however, was the opportunity for creativity and innovation. Kuhn provides considerably more openness for creativity by allowing some role for innovative puzzle solving particularly in responding to anomalies. Even for Kuhn, however, creativity is limited due to the parameters imposed by the paradigm. This could be considered a significant problem in a discipline such as nursing in view of its diverse and multifaceted focus and the dynamic nature of human beings and health situations. Innovation and creativity may be important in such a field and likely in any science.

---

[1]See especially the work of Sir Karl Popper (1959, 1963) and Imre Lakatos (1978).

BOX 7-2

MAJOR POINTS OF KUHN'S HISTORICISM

- Science is puzzle-solving.
- Science is organized around paradigms.
- Normal science is focused on articulating and expanding the paradigm.
- Anomalies develop, and if not accounted for by the paradigm, can accumulate and lead to crisis.
- New paradigm emerges and normal science results following crisis.
- Science is cumulative and linear to the crisis stage.
- Products of science must be evaluated relative to the paradigm.

DEMARCATION OF SCIENCE AND NONSCIENCE

Another significant aspect of Kuhn's work is the fact that he did not differentiate science from nonscience on the basis of subject matter or methods of inquiry. These aspects of science were determined in regard to the particular paradigm guiding the inquiry. Science, then, becomes a matter of process and activity rather than content and criteria. The focus on paradigms, which include methods and exemplars appropriate to the paradigm, allows greater flexibility in the types of inquiry and the specific methods that might be used in the work of "science."

This flexibility was a far better fit with the interests of nurse researchers. Since the facts, phenomena, theories, and hypotheses appropriate to science were freed from the rigid restrictions of the hypothetico-deductive approach, nurses had much more range for addressing phenomena relevant to the discipline. Nursing research could include, for example, a variety of methods depending on the needs and interests of the community of nurse scientists. Kuhn did not provide much detail, however, to resolve questions about whether or not multiple paradigms could exist simultaneously. A singular paradigm serving to direct all research activities in a discipline would exclude scientists in a field from working on unique and unrelated problems in very different ways. An immediate example that comes to mind concerns the very different types of problems addressed by researchers using qualitative methods and how such work might coexist with more traditional science. In the field of medicine (as in all health care actually), it is difficult to see how Kuhn's views would explain the simultaneous existence of work focused on genetic, biochemical, and "germ" origins of disease. According to Kuhn's viewpoint, a paradigm serves as a disciplinary matrix and would need to account for all the work in the discipline. Such diverse viewpoints involving different methods, theories, and phenomena can and do exist within disciplines and can direct the attention of researchers at the same time.

In spite of this significant limitation of Kuhn's view, scholars in nursing wrote extensively about the relevance of Kuhn's views for the development of nursing knowledge. References to Kuhn's work on scientific revolutions were common in the theoretical literature of nursing in the 1970s and 1980s and the term "paradigm" quickly became imbedded in the vocabulary of nursing science. As a result of comparing the status of nursing to "science" as described by Kuhn, writers in nursing tended to assess nursing as being at the preparadigm stage of development. As has been the case with many philosophies available during nursing's earlier scholarly period (the 1970s and 1980s particularly), the philosophy was used as a model of science and was considered to provide criteria for evaluation of the scientific status of nursing. Assessed according to Kuhn's position, nursing was determined to have an established "metaparadigm" but not the clear paradigm called for in Kuhn's philosophy. Kim (1989) did identify some paradigms used in nursing, noting the frequent use of concepts from General Systems Theory, Behaviorism, Phenomenology, and a few others. She saw research conducted using such ideas, however, as being based on the combination of multiple perspectives and not derived from a single "paradigm" to guide research in nursing. She observed subsequently that significant paradigms might emerge from these seemingly disparate viewpoints. Many nurse authors seemed to imply that such convergence of ideas into paradigms was essential for scientific progress to occur in nursing, indicating a general acceptance of Kuhn's viewpoint at least for awhile.

Hardy, who wrote extensively on the nature of theory in nursing in the 1970s and 1980s, provides a particularly clear example of the influence of Kuhn's work on philosophy of science and on the development of the knowledge base of nursing. Hardy earlier had shown the strong influence of the Received View formulation of science that had been popular at the time and was evident in the disciplines in which many nurse scholars had been educated. In a later article, however, Hardy (1983) cited Kuhn extensively; although discussing metaparadigms particularly, she proceeded to give considerable credence to Kuhn's views as appropriate for nursing.

Over time as nurses became more familiar with philosophy and philosophical principles included in educational programs, the limitations of Kuhn's view became more apparent. Kuhn's focus on paradigms and disciplinary matrices did not match much of what had occurred in the history of science. Kuhn's philosophy thus failed at a descriptive level. Numerous questions were raised as well regarding whether or not Kuhn's view could serve as a model for scientific development. One significant question addressed the possibility of multiple paradigms and the limitations of cumulative processes in scientific progress. Although Kuhn did break away from the strictly cumulative and linear approach of the Logical Positivists, the process of normal science described by Kuhn does reflect some remnants of this approach. From a standpoint of disciplinary identity, it was not clear how disciplines maintained any sense of continuity through time. If paradigms underwent change in a revolutionary manner, what held the discipline together and gave it a focus or purpose through all this change? These are some of the questions and challenges raised by later historicists.

LAUDAN'S VIEW OF SCIENCE

Larry Laudan, another prominent philosopher in the historicist tradition, presented a view of science similar to that of Kuhn in many ways. This is to be expected because both philosophers are grounded in a similar philosophical tradition. In other words, all Historicist philosophers, just as all Positivist philosophers, show considerable similarity in their positions in regard to major tenets of their philosophies. One area of similarity for Laudan and Kuhn is evident in Laudan's use of the phrase **problem-solving** to describe the primary activity of science, a phrase that bears very close resemblance to Kuhn's "puzzle-solving." Beyond this striking similarity, there are a number of important differences in the views of these two philosophers.

Critique of Kuhn's View

Although Laudan and Kuhn both focus on the processes of science and share an interest in the contextual aspects of scientific progress, Laudan describes numerous problems with Kuhn's view. First Laudan argues that it is rare for one paradigm to achieve the dominance evident in Kuhn's philosophy. In contrast to Kuhn's depiction of "normal science," the "revolutions" really are more normal according to Laudan. Disharmony is the persistent aspect of science with a "perennial coexistence of conflicting traditions" (Laudan, 1977, p. 136) being the norm rather than the unified approach depicted by Kuhn's reliance on a single paradigm to guide the work of scientists.

Laudan also argued against Kuhn's idea of the "incommensurability" of paradigms. Kuhn described the decision process when competing paradigms existed as a matter of judgment. Because the paradigm influences the scientists' perspectives so extensively and the scientific work conducted similarly reflects the influence of the paradigm, it is not possible simply to compare one paradigm to another in regard to its truth value or accuracy. In other words, scientists might prefer to follow the paradigm that is more "right," but it is not possible to make this determination due to the influence of the paradigm on all aspects of scientific activity. This difference in perspective and the inability to compare one paradigm to another in a direct manner is the basis of the "incommensurability" problem in science.

Laudan points out, however, that the concern with incommensurability is not relevant to determining future direction for scientific pursuits. The question for scientists is not really one of which paradigm is more "accurate" or more "true." In addition, incommensurability is a concern only when one paradigm is compared directly to another; yet the decision scientists typically face is not a decision of choosing one single paradigm among competing paradigms. Laudan argues, instead, that different approaches to science should be evaluated on their "problem-solving" effectiveness and contribution to progress, a situation that does not require direct comparison among approaches.

Problem Solving

For Laudan, the basis for scientific activity is "progress" with effectiveness in solving problems being the key to evaluating different approaches to scientific work. Where Kuhn described science as a "puzzle-solving" activity, Laudan focuses on problems as a more specific variant of Kuhn's emphasis. For Laudan, continuity in the sciences is provided through the problems addressed by the scientists not through the succession of revolutions and paradigm changes described by Kuhn. Laudan also faulted Kuhn for failing to give attention and weight to conceptual problems in science. The procedures used by scientists would be dictated by the paradigm to some extent; yet the emphasis throughout Kuhn's text is on empirical problems with little mention of the conceptual realm of scientific activity.

RESEARCH TRADITIONS

Laudan (1977) organizes the problem-solving activity of science into "research traditions" in contrast to Kuhn's paradigms. Laudan defines a **research tradition** as "a set of general assumptions about the entities and processes in a domain of study and about the appropriate methods to be used for investigating the problems and constructing the theories in that domain" (p. 81). A research tradition includes assumptions about phenomena and methods and theories relevant to the tradition. In contrast to Kuhn's view in which the entire paradigm changes through a process of revolution, Laudan points out how any part of the research tradition can change. Laudan sees research traditions as continually evolving over time rather than undergoing a sweeping change. In this sense, Laudan is consistent with other philosophers, including Stephen Toulmin (see Chapter 8), who take an evolutionary view of the development of science.

This idea of research traditions provides the basis for Laudan's exploration of rationality and scientific progress. According to Laudan, a broader notion of rationality is needed than that presented by the Logical Positivists, which showed rationality as driven by clear criteria of Truth. Laudan (1977) argues, in contrast, for the inclusion of seemingly "non-scientific" factors (p. 132) as legitimate components of rationality. Laudan redefined rationality as acting to "do whatever we can to maximize the progress of scientific research traditions" (p. 124). Rationality, according to Laudan, is not based on a specific singular goal or criterion of truth, for example, but simply on maximizing the progress of scientific work. What exactly counts as progress is the solving of problems. According to Laudan, the progress of a research tradition is a function of problem-solving adequacy and the speed with which progress is occurring. Laudan initially presents his concern with evaluating the adequacy of a research tradition in a very concise formula: The number of empirical problems solved minus the number of conceptual and anomalous problems generated = Problem-solving effectiveness.

This formula may seem overly simplistic and it is on first reading. Evaluation of a research tradition, however, is not merely a matter of counting the number of problems solved or generated. Laudan instead provides a detailed system of weighting problems that places greater significance on particular types of problems.

ASSIGNING WEIGHT TO PROBLEMS

Weighting of problems is an important part of Laudan's philosophy. This evaluation of problem solving is relative to the research traditions that exist at the time and compete for attention, support, and resources. Evaluation of problem-solving effectiveness also is relative to previous theories that exist within the research tradition as well as to prevailing doctrines for theory assessment.

Bearing in mind all these considerations, scientists give different weight to problems according to numerous factors. Increased weight is given to a problem, for example, that has been solved previously; in other words, an alternative theory needs to account for solved problems in addition to anything else new it might offer. Problems that have presented anomalies and resisted solution also will be given increased weight as their resistance to solution increases their value and consideration. Some problems serve as particularly outstanding examples in a science, constituting a sort of archetype form of problems. These types of problems warrant special consideration and higher weighting as well. Finally additional weight may be given to problems of great generality such that a solution for the problem also provides a solution for a number of previous problems. Solutions to such problems include solutions to an array of problems in the field.

CONCEPTUAL PROBLEMS

It is important to note that while Laudan emphasizes empirical problems, he gives considerable attention to conceptual problems as well. Laudan (1977) points out that "it would be an enormous mistake, however, to imagine that scientific progress and rationality consist entirely of solving empirical problems" (p. 45). Laudan further describes conceptual problem solving as "at least as important in the development of science" (p. 45) as empirical problem solving. Laudan devotes an entire chapter of his book to conceptual problems in an effort to "state the case for a richer theory of problem solving than empiricists have allowed, to explore the nature of these nonempirical problems and show what role they have in theory appraisal" (p. 45). Laudan contends that conceptual problems have played a significant role in science throughout history. The typical response of scientists, however, "has been to deplore the intrusion of these 'unscientific' considerations" (p. 47). In contrast to such a response, Laudan attempts to incorporate such aspects into a general scheme of science.

A **conceptual problem**, according to Laudan (1977), is "a *problem exhibited by some theory or other*" (italics in original). Conceptual problems are "characteristics of theories and have no existence independent of the theories which exhibit them" (p. 48). They may be *internal* to a theory, in which case the theory demonstrates internal inconsistency, or external, as evident when theories are in conflict (p. 49). Laudan provides considerably more detail on the nature of such problems. For purposes here, it is most important to note Laudan's emphasis on conceptual problems in addition to empirical problems in science. He disagrees strongly with "scholars (such as Kuhn) [who] have gone so far as to make the absence of such nonempirical factors a token of the 'maturity' of any specific science" (p. 47). For Laudan, it is clear that conceptual problems must be attended to along with the empirical problems confronted in a science.

In addition to questioning this position on the role of conceptual problems in the determination of a science as "mature" or not, Laudan challenges the notion of mature and immature science on a broader level. The evolution of science does not reveal that the transition to a mature science is a permanent one, particularly in regard to achieving maturity as a result of the dominant role of a single paradigm. Laudan also questions the position of Kuhn and Lakatos that mature sciences "would be intrinsically more progressive and more scientific than 'immature' ones" (Laudan, 1977, p. 151). Finally he argues that the idea of mature versus immature is in a sense self-validating as the "models are chiefly designed as replicas of 'mature science'" (p. 151). In other words, a science is purported to be mature and criteria consistent with that science are put forth as examples of a mature science. This makes it possible to dismiss examples that do not fit the model of mature science. It is common to label such sciences as "pseudoscience." Laudan acknowledges that a model of mature science might be found eventually; presently though, it offers little to an effort to understand how science functions and progresses (p. 151).

Laudan and the Sociology of Knowledge

The conclusion of Laudan's (1977) view in the text, *Progress and Its Problems*, is a detailed discussion of how Laudan applies his ideas to understanding the history of science with a glimpse of the sociological aspects of knowledge as well. Consistent with a Historicist position, Laudan points out the intricate relationship between the work of knowledge development and the institutional and organizational structures associated with that work. He poses an extensive challenge to prevailing ideas of a sociology of knowledge, however, finding them to be based on false assumptions about science and rationality and the inability to associate scientific developments with social structures and beliefs in the case of cognitive sociology. According to Laudan, this focus in the sociology of knowledge "is predicated on the existence of determinable correlations between the social background of a scientist and the specific belief about the physical world which he [sic] espouses" (p. 217). This statement seems to recognize the emerging postmodern trends of the time (see Chapter 9) in which science is associated with themes such as classism, sexism, and domination and oppression. Laudan clearly rejects that science necessarily involves such a perspective, emphasizing that it is the practice of cognitive sociology in regard to science that he opposes and not the idea of such a sociology of science.

Laudan instead points out the many areas in his own work that lend themselves well to greater sociological understanding, the weighting of problems, and the acceptance of a research tradition that seems less progressive than another as just two examples in which sociological illumination would be welcomed (p. 224). Ultimately he purports that the effort to understand the world is an inherent quality of humans. Organized around Research Traditions, scientists are able to judge and give priority to significant problems and to work on both theoretical and conceptual levels. Scientists are challenged to focus on relevant and significant problems and follow a sufficiently progressive path worthy of the resources "lavished" upon them.

With the possibility of multiple research traditions existing within a science (or discipline), this organizational structure provides greater flexibility and enables varied foci of interest to occupy the work of a science at any particular time. Empirical problems continue to be emphasized but not to the exclusion of other types of problems. The emphasis on problem solving alone carries a sense of pragmatism or usefulness. Although the science may determine its relevant problems through the lens of its own knowledge needs, the opportunity to look at problems from a broader standpoint of application fits easily with those needs. Through such an approach, Laudan provides a view of science that is broader and more flexible, problem-focused, and relevant while still recognizing the importance of rational processes and progress.

Laudan's Contributions to Science and Nursing

Laudan provides a very practical and applied view of science. His focus on problem solving, balance of conceptual and empirical problems, and emphasis on "relevance" in regard to truth characterize his position as a stark contrast to some of the earlier views of science and perhaps to the mainstream idea of science as well. This pragmatic position seems an excellent fit with the nursing goals and purposes focused on providing meaningful interventions to promote health. Laudan, in fact, notes that "the workability of the problem-solving model is its greatest virtue" (p. 127). With this view, it is possible to determine whether or not science is progressive and rational, criteria that must be met to understand the activities of scientists and to promote scientific progress. Work occurs on both the empirical and the conceptual levels, and priority can be assigned to problems according to a variety of factors including importance, length of time the problem has confronted the science, and comprehensiveness or generality of the problem.

In addition to these general characteristics of Laudan's view (see Box 7-3), the organization of science into Research Traditions allows greater flexibility and vari-

BOX 7-3·

MAJOR POINTS OF LAUDAN'S HISTORICISM

- ◆ Science is problem solving.
- ◆ Science involves both empirical and conceptual problems.
- ◆ Weighting of problems determines priority and importance.
- ◆ Science is organized around research traditions.
- ◆ Multiple Research Traditions can exist in a field or discipline.
- ◆ Knowledge claims need to be evaluated relative to the research tradition.

ety within a scientific field. Unlike Kuhn's notion of a paradigm that constitutes a "matrix" for the discipline, Laudan's discussion of Research Traditions does not exclude the possibility of multiple traditions existing simultaneously in a discipline. Laudan describes a process by which separate traditions can be integrated and a scientist actually may work in more than one research tradition at a time. In nursing, a situation of this type is occurring with the blending of community health concepts with content from other forms of nursing as nurses become increasingly cognizant of the role of environments and context in relation to human health. As with all scientific development, this process of "amalgamation" of separate traditions occurs in an evolutionary rather than a revolutionary manner, according to Laudan.

Laudan, as well as Kuhn, places considerable emphasis on values and ideals in the activities of science. In a subsequent text, *Science and Values*, Laudan (1984) focuses more specifically on the role of values and acknowledges how consensus typically is difficult to generate. In contrast, dissent can stimulate scientific work and promote discussion; it is not essential to have agreement on values before work can progress or rationality can be determined.

Fry (1995) claims that Laudan's work "can be a powerful model for nursing science" (p. 79) and recommends that his approach "receive serious consideration" (p. 80). His work addresses many shortcomings of Kuhn's philosophy and certainly those of the Received View; Laudan's work has received consideration and support from numerous authors in nursing (Kegly, 1995; Thompson, 1985; Tinkle & Beaton,1983). Laudan is particularly significant for the work of nurse scientists for several reasons including his emphasis on "problem-solving." In view of the applied or practical focus of the work of nursing, this way of framing knowledge development seems more tenable than seeking Truth. Nurses also work with the very complex subject matter of humans and health. This content can be viewed from a variety of perspectives including physical, psychological, behavioral, social, affective, and aesthetic. Working with such complex phenomena in a comprehensive and meaningful manner requires that nurses have a view of science that allows for a variety of forms of inquiry consistent with the problem being addressed in the inquiry. Laudan's approach, which supports the existence of multiple Research Traditions in a field that still maintains some identity as a discipline, is worthy of consideration for nursing science.

CONCLUSION

Regardless of the utility of future application of the work of either Kuhn or Laudan, there can be no question that Historicism provides a new perspective on the position, role, and procedures of science, the determination of progress, and the nature of a discipline. Both of these philosophers introduce ideas presumed to be separate from science, particularly such ideas as values, consensus, and judgment, and the fact that science is an act of scientists rather than merely a body of knowledge. With their perspectives, students of science and philosophy are encouraged to view science as a human enterprise rather than a knowledge product that takes a particular form. The compelling arguments provided for consideration of the human component of science must be addressed in attempts to understand and promote further development of nursing science.

FOR DISCUSSION

1. Describe the major tenets of the historicist views of Kuhn and Laudan.
2. Compare and contrast Logical Positivism and historicism as philosophies of science. Consider as part of this discussion the goals, procedures, and criteria for evaluating progress in science as presented in each view.
3. Discuss the implications of a focus on process versus product as a means to evaluate science.
4. Discuss similarities and differences in the historicist position and the development of nursing science.
5. Identify examples of empirical and conceptual problems in nursing inquiry.
6. Identify examples of paradigms and/or research traditions in nursing.

REFERENCES

Fry, S. T. (1995). Science as problem solving. In A. Omery, C. E. Kasper, & G. G. Page, (Eds.), *In search of nursing science* (pp. 72–80). Thousand Oaks, CA: Sage.

Hardy, M. (1983). Metaparadigms and theory development. In N. L. Chaska (Ed.), *The nursing profession: A time to speak* (pp. 427–437). New York: McGraw-Hill.

Kegly, J. A. K. (1995). Science as tradition and tradition shattering. In A. Omery, C. E. Kasper, & G. G. Page, (Eds.), *In search of nursing science* (pp. 43–57). Thousand Oaks, CA: Sage.

Kim, H. S. (1989). Theoretical thinking in nursing: Problems and prospects. *Recent Advances in Nursing, 24,* 106–122.

Kuhn, T. S. (1970). *The structure of scientific revolutions* (2 ed.). Chicago: University of Chicago. (originally published 1962).

Kuhn, T. S. (1974). Second thoughts on paradigms. In F. Suppe (Ed.), *The structure of scientific theories* (pp. 459–482). Urbana: University of Illinois.

Kuhn, T. S. (1977). *The essential tension: Selected studies in scientific tradition and change.* Chicago: University of Chicago Press.

Lakatos, I. (1978). *The methodology of scientific research programmes.* Cambridge: Cambridge University Press.

Laudan, L. (1977). *Progress and its problems.* Berkeley: University of California Press.

Laudan, L. (1984). *Science and values.* Berkeley: University of California.

Popper, K. (1959). *Logic of scientific discovery.* New York: Basic Books.

Popper, K. (1963). *Conjectures and refutations.* London: Routledge & Kegan Paul.

Thompson, J. (1985). Practical discourse in nursing: Going beyond empiricism and historicism. *Advances in Nursing Science, 7*(4), 59–71.

Tinkle, M. B., & Beaton, J. L. (1983). Toward a new view of science: Implications for nursing research. *Advances in Nursing Science, 5*(2), 27–36.

Conceptual Repertoires and Leaps

As a philosophy of science, Historicism places an emphasis on processes and contexts as the means to understand scientific activity. The work of Stephen Toulmin presents an interesting variation on Historicist philosophy of science. Drawing specifically on the principles of evolution presented by Charles Darwin (1859), Toulmin's work demonstrates what can be referred to as an evolutionary perspective. Toulmin's philosophy offers much more than just a position on the activities of scientists and their construction of knowledge and is not merely substituting "evolution" for the "revolution" in Kuhn's view. A greater appreciation of Toulmin's contributions can be gained by stepping back briefly to revisit the development of epistemology in general over the past several centuries.

BACKGROUNDS FOR UNDERSTANDING TOULMIN

Precedence of the Rational View of Science

For most of the 20th century, philosophers of science were occupied with constructing a rational view of science and scientific progress. A **rational** view allows analysis of science on the basis of factors internal to the science rather than on contextual factors or factors external to the science. According to this view, a rational approach to science must explicate 1) the goal of science (most commonly, Truth), and 2) the means of evaluating or choosing between rival theories. Another way of stating this is that a rational view of science holds that science has a goal and that there are clear criteria for determining progress toward that goal. Rational science starts with a set of rules and follows an agreed-upon **heuristic**, or a guide for further inquiry, for continuing progress. The degree of rationality evident in the views presented by various philosophers of science represents a continuum rather than creating a situation in which a philosophy can be labeled simply as rational or non-rational.[1]

Kuhn's Influence on Rationalism in Science

Kuhn presented a challenge to the prevailing idea of Rationalism by introducing elements of context and of the scientists themselves into discussions of scientific progress. Kuhn pointed out that science has a history rather than an essence to be explored. Kuhn argued that he was not being relativist in his position, although the merits of this argument are questionable in view of the emphasis placed on history, context, and paradigms. Armed with the credibility provided through his background in theoretical physics, Kuhn brought a view of science as a dynamic enterprise; science could be understood best not by a static view but from a historical and moving account. Positions such as Kuhn's gave new meaning to the idea of rationality: rationality lies in the procedures governing its historical development and change rather than in a single logical system.

---

[1]In recent years, attempts to construct strictly rational views of science have been less common. Part of the reason for leaving this approach was that such attempts have been unsuccessful for the most part in the context of modern science. Philosophers had great difficulty developing a view of science that adequately explained progress by focusing on the scientific enterprise alone, in other words, on the internal workings of science. Paul Feyerabend (1975), in his popular text *Against Method*, viewed science as somewhat arbitrary and ideologically based, pointing out the importance of recognizing the role of beliefs in science. His position for what is most appropriate in science was summarized as "anything goes," particularly valuing creativity and novelty in scientific activity. His work was criticized heavily for a number of reasons not the least of which was the fact that his views were not at all agreeable to those who believed that science was or should be rational in its activities.

This view of science has a great deal of appeal, providing reason and justification for looking at both history and context when examining science. Nurses certainly would not consider clients or patients, the people around them, or the current status of nursing without some concern for what had taken place before. It is highly questionable, then, why science should be devoid of such consideration.

As appealing as the concern with history may be there are some problems with Kuhn's and similar positions. One of the most significant limitations of Kuhn's position is that the history of science does not fit his revolutionary scenario. For example, Kuhn gives the impression that the change from classical physics of Newton and Galileo to the relativity theory of Einstein represents a more or less unconscious progression or change in world view, that earlier theories were more or less overthrown as a result of a great and sudden awareness of what was more accurate. In contrast, Kuhn's own historical analysis of the change from pre-Copernican astronomy to the science of Newton and Galileo, which he described in *The Copernican Revolution* (1957), raises questions about the "revolutionary" nature of this shift. Kuhn's own account shows that this change took nearly a century and a half to complete and was subject to considerable debate at every turn. The change ultimately occurred because the arguments were there to convince astronomers not because the old views were discounted or because scientists were compelled by their peers to adopt the new view. This situation, in general, seems a poor fit with the idea of revolutions put forth by Kuhn.

What remains is that paradigm changes may not be as complete as Kuhn's approach implies. Rival paradigms also may not amount to completely alternative world views. While there are certainly discontinuities on the theoretical level of science, continuities remain on other levels such as with methodological aspects. Focusing only on the changes that occur and not the continuities that persist may overlook a large component of scientific progress. As noted in Chapter 7, Kuhn's view may explain partly why scientists pursue the avenues they choose to explore but it does not explain what provides the continuity in the science.

 ## TOULMIN'S IDEA OF SCIENCE

Laudan raised this question about continuity as well, identifying that problems provide continuity in the science. Similarly Toulmin looks at the development of science in a manner that recognizes both continuity and change in the process of scientific progress. These observations provide some background for Toulmin's (1972) *Human Understanding*. Some issues raised by Toulmin include factors that contribute to change; even if complete paradigm changes do not occur, certainly there is some change and Toulmin questions what accounts for that change as well as how dissent and consensus occur. Toulmin also questions what accounts for the underlying consistencies that remain despite some change and identifies the need to explain how progress should be viewed. Finally he identifies the problem of separating the practice of knowledge from its theory, in other words, separating science from epistemology. Are scientists merely those who do science as the passive recipients of progressive changes or are they essential elements that must be considered if we are to talk intelligently about the nature of science?

Inward-Looking Versus Outward-Looking Approaches

In response to these questions, Toulmin (1972) aims to construct a new "epistemic self-portrait" (p. 25), which he describes as "a fresh account of the capacities, processes, and activities, in virtue of which Man (sic) acquires an understanding of Nature, and Nature, in turn, becomes intelligible to Man (sic)" (p. 25). Toulmin's position can be understood better by looking at one other aspect of discussion in western philosophy of science. Since the 1600s or so, philosophers tended to take one of two slants in examining epistemology. These can be referred to simplistically as "inward looking" or "outward looking" (p. 3) approaches to knowledge. An inward-looking view, according to Toulmin, is philosophical or theoretical in origin and addresses the standards used in making judgments about knowledge (p. 3). In another sense, inward-looking epistemologies might be viewed as focused on examining the workings of the human mind or human cognition. An outward-looking view concerns practical standards and the application of judgments about knowledge claims. It might also be thought of as looking to the nature of the external world and how it is constituted so that knowledge can reflect or capture it properly. On an epistemic level, Empiricism is a prime example of an outward-looking view; for most of the 20th century, the emphasis has been on such externally focused activities particularly in the pursuit of Truth about the external world.

At the same time, philosophers have dealt with the problems of knowledge and understanding on a primarily individual level. From John Locke to Bertrand Russell, orthodox epistemologists have interpreted the problem of knowledge as the need to explain, first, how an individual thinker can arrive at valid ideas or truths. Only recently has there been much attempt to connect individual knowledge with the social realm of existence. Ludwig Wittgenstein likely had an influential role in this change due to his work that stimulated an emphasis on the role of language in the development of knowledge. Perhaps Descartes also provided a foundation for the persistence of this dilemma between inward-looking and outward-looking approaches as a result of his distinction between the mind and physical bodies, or the inner mind and the external world (sometimes referred to as the private-public distinction).

Toulmin is faced with the problem of how to penetrate private experience so as to describe or construct an external world of public objects that exist beyond that private experience. Toulmin's question is not one of just knowledge but of understanding, the grasping or "penetration" of knowledge in the human mind. Toulmin's attempt at a holistic approach is not a totally new idea in philosophy but in recent years it has undergone much development. Hans Reichenbach introduced the idea in 1938 in his book *Experience and Prediction*. In this work, Reichenbach introduced the phrases "context of discovery" and "context of justification" into philosophical discussion. This idea of looking at the context in which science takes place has been referred to as **Weltanschauungen** analyses, using a term from German to capture the comprehensive (holistic) nature of the view. This type of work is not new to Toulmin either; he presented a similar form of analysis in opposition to the Received View in an earlier text on the philosophy of science (Toulmin, 1953). Weltanschauungen analyses go beyond the traditional inward- versus outward-looking approaches; they typically involve attention to a variety of factors associated with the knowledge-generating enterprise particularly the common bonds of language and methodology.

Concepts

Regardless of the philosopher's type of analysis, one feature is common to nearly all discussions. A central term involved in nearly all discussions of knowledge and understanding, what might be considered a tool of knowledge, is the notion of **concept**. Considerable confusion exists regarding what a concept is; this confusion has presented a significant impediment to development of an effective portrait of science. Attention to concepts has been so great throughout epistemology and philosophy of science that it provides a focus for differentiating philosophical views and tracing progression in thought over time.

It is no surprise that Toulmin also incorporates content about concepts in his discussion. Toulmin goes well beyond the mere mention or recognition of concepts, however, as he builds his entire philosophical system on his ideas about concepts and their role in science. Toulmin (1972) indicates that his first concern is to

> consider concepts as entering into the conceptual aggregates, systems, or populations that are employed on a collective basis by communities of 'concept users.' We can concern ourselves with the patterns of events through which such aggregates of concepts are created, develop historically, and fall into disuse; and ask in what respects the resulting changes—historical or sociological, anthropological or whatever—have a bearing on the intellectual authority of the concepts concerned. (p.12)

Beyond looking at what concepts are and what can be done with them, Toulmin extends his concern to how certain concepts, or a system of concepts, become established and gain authority in a discipline. This includes attention not only to the patterns of concept development and change but also to the sociological aspects of the "concept users" that provide the context for such activity.

Toulmin's framework for a foundation for his inquiry into conceptual change is derived from Darwin's work on evolution and the principles of variation and selective perpetuation (natural selection) (Toulmin, 1972, p. 135). Toulmin employs the principles of Darwin as a form of general historical explanation, providing useful insights into how change occurs over time. Toulmin argues that this idea of evolution can be applied to all historical entities—people, institutions, and even knowledge development (p. 135). Before exploring Toulmin's idea of concepts in more depth, understanding his approach to the organization of sciences is useful background for his ideas because certain conditions must be satisfied for the principles of Darwin's work to be relevant.

Definitions of a Discipline

According to Toulmin (1972), a **discipline** is characterized in regard to three interrelated elements: "(i) the current explanatory goals of the science, (ii) its current repertory of concepts and procedures, and (iii) the accumulated experience of the scientists working in the particular discipline" (p. 175). In contrast, a **profession** is an "organized set of institutions, roles, and [people] whose business it is to apply or improve the procedures and techniques" of the discipline (p. 142). In this view, discipline and profession are inseparable. Without a profession to continue to use and develop the knowledge contained in the discipline, a discipline would not progress or change and ultimately would cease to exist. Toulmin seems to be saying that knowledge has little real value without people to use and develop it. This also seems to indicate that knowledge, created, perpetuated, and disseminated by people has an inherent social aspect to its existence. Toulmin does not provide great detail about the relationship between a discipline and a profession; this leaves some questions about whether there is one profession for each discipline or if several professions exist and share the knowledge of a discipline. Regardless of these lingering questions, however, it is clear that for Toulmin the members of a profession work with the knowledge, procedures, and techniques of the discipline.

In keeping with a focus on the human and social structuring of disciplines, Toulmin provides additional detail about how disciplines develop. The crucial element in a discipline, according to Toulmin, is recognition of a sufficiently agreed upon goal or ideal in terms of which common outstanding problems can be identified. Scientific disciplines are delineated by having "explanatory" goals or ideals, in other words, a focus on providing explanation of things that exist in the world (p. 364). Focused around this ideal, disciplines can develop in ways that resemble a continuum of organization and clarity. **Compact disciplines** meet criteria of being organized; they have clearly stated goals, established professional forums, and agreement on criteria of adequacy when evaluating explanations and knowledge developments. Toulmin applies the terms **diffuse** and **would-be disciplines** to more loosely structured disciplines. Disciplines that function in this manner fail to meet the criteria of a compact discipline on either methodological or institutional levels. As Toulmin describes it, "one of the best indications that a new science has arrived at a clear definition of its intellectual goals, and achieved a proper disciplinary status, is the eventual enthronement of an agreed set of fundamental concepts and selection criteria" (p. 381). A discipline, therefore, must exhibit some intellectual ideals, some things the discipline desires to explain or understand.

Toulmin's Definition of Scientific Problems

This notion of disciplines is important in examining Toulmin's work and certainly of relevance and interest in nursing (see Box 8-1). Whether or not any discipline demonstrates characteristics consistent with a "compact" or a "would-be" or "diffuse" state of existence, Toulmin's views are still applicable to the study of scientific progress and change. Recognition of the fundamental role of explanatory ideals to a science and the focus of scientific work on identified problems are central to studying this process. Toulmin defines scientific problems using a very simple formula:

scientific problems = explanatory ideals - current capacities (p. 152)

As evident in this formula, Toulmin displays some similarity to Laudan in that they both see problems as a focus of scientific activity and the evaluation of progress. For Toulmin, problems serve as the stimulus for change with a goal of science being to solve problems, thereby, increasing movement toward accomplishing the intellectual ideals of the discipline.

This formula, along with Toulmin's discussion of the context of scientific activity, provides a foundation for understanding how science progresses. As Toulmin describes it, the intellectual ideals provide a connection among the various elements of the discipline. Initially a discipline may not have a clear focus in regard to its appropriate goals and procedures. As it evolves, the goals become more clear

---

BOX 8-1

SCIENTIFIC PROBLEMS AND NURSING

Toulmin's idea of scientific problems has relevance throughout nursing. For purposes of illustration, consider the intriguing challenge presented by persons who do well, who thrive and achieve in spite of incredible challenges. Nursing has a repertoire of concepts such as coping and adaptation that help to explain part of this situation. Yet an understanding is lacking about how some people are able not only to overcome but also to grow as a result of adversity. The explanatory ideal of understanding the mechanisms that underlie resilience or inner strength and being able to support these positive occurrences is not met through current capacities in regard to coping and adaptation. The result is a scientific problem associated with this positive health phenomenon possibly related to a different concept of resilience.

and specific and there is the development of some agreement about the explanatory procedures relevant to those goals. Those explanatory procedures are inextricably linked to the conceptual base of the discipline. The concepts are the focus of scientific effort to address problems. The concepts of the discipline provide historical continuity; they form a "**transmit**" (p. 158) of content that is passed on from one generation of scientists to the next through a process of "**enculturation**" (p. 159). In a form of apprenticeship, explanatory skills embodied in the concepts are conveyed through successive generations.

Understanding the Concepts of a Discipline

LEVELS AND IMPORTANCE OF RESOLVING CONCEPTUAL PROBLEMS

In gaining an understanding the discipline's concepts, Toulmin (1972) describes how the new scientist must understand that concepts possess several levels of importance. Work to resolve conceptual problems takes place on three levels and concerns separate yet related aspects of concepts. Perhaps the most obvious level for work on conceptual problems concerns the language with which concepts are communicated. This "linguistic" component involves both the terminology (or names) applied to concepts and sentences employing those names.

Representation techniques, according to Toulmin (1972), constitute another aspect of concepts that may be addressed in attempts to resolve conceptual problems. These techniques include "all those varied procedures by which scientists demonstrate—i.e., exhibit, rather than prove deductively—the general relations discoverable among natural objects, events and phenomena..." (p. 162). These representation techniques include various ways of illustrating the concepts including mathematical forms, graphs, diagrams, classification systems, and computer programs (p. 162).

Along with the component of language, the representation techniques constitute the "symbolic" aspects of concepts. There must be clear criteria concerning the application of the concepts for the concepts to have any meaning in the science. Scientists must be able to determine what situations warrant application of the concept and the situations in which the concepts do not apply. Without understanding the "'scope' or 'range of application'" of the concepts, they may have no "empirical relevance" for the scientists (p. 162). In attempts to resolve conceptual problems, some combination of language, representation techniques, and application procedures is involved and must be addressed.

In the history of the philosophy of science, empirical problems have received far more attention than problems of a conceptual nature. In fact in view of the origins of science in empiricism, it is likely that most people think of science primarily if not exclusively in regard to its empirical orientation. Even Kuhn pointed out that the empirical success of a new paradigm contributes to its continuing progress and revolution.

Toulmin, like Laudan (1977), gives considerable attention to the role of conceptual problems in science. Laudan, however, treats empirical and conceptual problems essentially as two different classes of problems and gives each type equal consideration in evaluating theories. According to Laudan, overall problem-solving effectiveness is determined by assessing the number and importance of empirical problems solved and deducting from that the number and importance of anomalies and conceptual problems generated. Although empirical problems serve as the foundation of this equation (start with empirical problems solved and subtract from there), it is clear how anomalies and conceptual problems separately or together can detract significantly from the effectiveness of a theory. Toulmin, in contrast, presents a philosophy focused primarily on conceptual problems. For Toulmin, scientific activity is a process of concept development. Conceptual problems are resolved through work on both empirical and conceptual levels.

TYPES OF CONCEPTUAL PROBLEMS

Toulmin also is similar to Laudan in his position that conceptual problems are a critical focus of the work of science. Toulmin, however, has a more extensive list of the types of conceptual problems and he identifies five categories of problems (see Box 8-2). First, there are phenomena that a science reasonably expects to explain but currently has no procedure for working with the phenomena successfully. Conceptual problems also exist in a form where phenomena are partially accounted for but the understanding of the phenomenon is incomplete. Different concepts coexisting within a single branch of science may be a source of problems as well or there may be conflicts between concepts in different fields of science; in other words, concepts are defined or applied differently in distinct disciplines. As the final type of conceptual problem addressed, Toulmin gives striking acknowledgment of the relationship between science and the public or society at large. He identifies as a separate category of conceptual problems the conflicts that can exist between concepts and procedures within science and the attitudes current among society at large. Such "extra-scientific" ideas may have implications if not immediate relevance for scientific discussions. Ideas such as responsibility, freedom, and life and death may enter into discussions generating conceptual problems that at least affect the work of scientists even though they may not be addressed directly in inquiry.

Explanation of Change

In addition to describing the proper activities of science, philosophers of science also must explain how change occurs in science. Scientists do not follow the same lead or ideas indefinitely. Philosophers face a considerable challenge describing what ignites the change of allegiance in ideology in the course of the history of science as well as what maintains some continuity in the field. Toulmin, in a manner similar to Laudan, sees problems as forming the background for change. Problems

---

BOX 8-2

TYPES OF CONCEPTUAL PROBLEMS

- ◆ Phenomena scientists want to explain but lack procedures (e.g., spirituality).
- ◆ Phenomena only partially understood (e.g., spirituality, grief)
- ◆ Conflict among concepts within a single discipline (e.g., coping, adaptation)
- ◆ Conflict among concepts in different disciplines (e.g., health)
- ◆ Conflict among concepts and societal attitudes (e.g., health, compliance)

---

have a significant focus in regard to the fact that change occurs to meet the explanatory ideals of the science. Yet change does not occur in a vacuum, and Toulmin devotes a great deal of attention to the context in which change occurs. Influencing factors within this context can include internal or intellectual considerations along with external or sociological considerations. Internal considerations are related to the nature of the problem in that the problem should be viewed as having some possibility of resolution. Forums of discussion and competition need to exist because the discipline should be professionally organized in ways that permit novel ideas to be appraised and evaluated. According to Toulmin, another internal consideration concerns the "ripeness" of the problem. Techniques, ideas, instruments, and other tools need to be present to make the problem something suitable for scientists to address. Ripeness may also refer to the problem having sufficient internal significance for the scientists to view it as having sufficient priority to address.

External considerations in the conduct of science also have a profound influence on scientists' activities. Such considerations provide incentives and opportunities for work in particular areas or may put obstacles in the way of innovations and work in other realms. As Toulmin (1972) describes the relationship between the internal and external factors, "intellectual considerations thus focus the theorizing which social incentives make possible" (p. 221).

In assessing the merits of ideas, Toulmin describes a fairly straightforward approach to evaluate variations and innovations in concepts. His criteria are highly practical and contextual. Toulmin argues that evaluating variations is first a matter of comparison for relevance, precision, detail, and applicability. The standards of judgment in regard to these criteria are informal and express the current disciplinary ideals. Rarely, Toulmin adds, can the merits of a variant be stated or evaluated in simple terms. In other words, it is not possible in most circumstances to state simply that one concept is "better" than another is. Similarly there is no means to quantify or score the contributions of alternatives. Evaluation typically rests on a **"strategic consensus"** (p. 231). In describing this process of consensus, Toulmin provides an interesting discussion of how reference groups become established, in other words, some groups become more influential and serve as the ultimate judges in the science:

> A new concept, theory, or strategy...becomes an effective 'possibility'...only when it is taken seriously by influential members of the relevant profession, and it becomes fully 'established' only when it wins their positive endorsement. (p. 266)

With this statement, Toulmin makes explicit the power and the institutions that influence intellectual functions and the progression of knowledge. This "Old Guard" eventually is replaced by a subsequent generation (p. 266) through the ongoing competition among various facets of the profession in a social and political manner not at all resembling the systematic account proposed by many philosophers (p. 270).

The Nature and Role of Concepts

Toulmin's view on the nature and role of concepts in the performance of science takes a position between treating concepts as merely words or as real properties of objects. The first position, which is referred to as nominalism, puts a primary focus on words. A nominalist position would treat "green" as merely a name attached to some things that all share this common condition of being green. Realism, in contrast, is the idea that things are called "green" because of some intrinsic property they share, some quality of green. Green, in a realist position, is a real object or entity separate from being talked about using the term "green."

As the preceding discussion reveals, Toulmin holds that disciplines possess a repertoire of concepts that form a "transmit." This transmit is passed along through successive generations of scientists who learn how to use the terminology and procedures appropriate to the conceptual repertoire and to apply the concepts in their attempt to achieve the explanatory ideals of the discipline. The remaining question to be addressed concerns the process of conceptual change and ultimate scientific progress. In Toulmin's view, as in Darwin's, change "can be explained in terms of a single dual process of variation and selective perpetuation" (p. 136). For this process to yield viable new variants, however, further conditions must be satisfied. "Selective pressure" is necessary for the advantages of the new concept to be evident. Without serious competition, variants have no chance to win support over their rivals. In addition, the competition must not be too extensive, otherwise the variant becomes too spread out and will not take hold. Variants also must be sufficiently "well adapted" to be perpetuated, in other words, able to cope with the demands of the discipline (pp. 137–138).

Role of "Strategic Consensus"

Where Kuhn introduced anomalies as posing a considerable threat to current scientific work, Toulmin sees the constant interplay of new ideas and existing concepts in an evolutionary manner: scientific work takes place to expand and enhance the conceptual repertoire of the science, stronger (or more promising, or more useful) concepts are retained and the weaker ones fade. A "strategic consensus" (p. 231) determines the criteria appropriate for selecting among variants, Toulmin adds,

> the scientists will agree in their judgments on conceptual innovations, simply because this consensus decides for them what kinds of changes will fulfill the agreed intellectual goals of the science for the time being. (p. 231)

Toulmin defines Rationality as an attribute of the procedures by which such judgments are made. It "has its own 'courts' in which all clear-headed men with suitable experience are qualified to act as judges or jurors" (p. 95). The principles may vary depending on the environment or context because there are no universal criteria for rationality. In other words, rationality is contextual rather than based on a foundation such as Truth-seeking. Consistent with Toulmin's arguments throughout this text, the determination of rationality involves a "populational" view rather than a "systematic" analysis, which would consider rationality from the viewpoint of formal logic. Conceptual change can be considered rational to the extent that it meets the demands of the discipline or contributes "towards solving the everyday problems of dealing effectively and harmoniously with our fellow-men, animals, or inanimate objects, as the case may be" (p. 493).

 ## SUMMARY OF TOULMIN'S WORK

Toulmin provides a view of science that goes at least a step beyond that of Kuhn and Laudan in several respects. The connection with Historicism should be clear because Toulmin's view has a strong emphasis on context, directing as much attention to the organization and conduct of science as to its content. Toulmin provides insightful detail on the relationship between discipline and profession and an intriguing illustration of the variations possible as disciplines develop. This discussion of compact, diffuse, and would-be disciplines is more enlightening for nursing than merely describing a discipline as in the preparadigm stage, for Toulmin describes the process of development rather than making claims about the discipline's current status.

Toulmin and Laudan share an interesting perspective on the role of "explanatory ideals" (to use Toulmin's words). For Toulmin, however, sharing objectives or goals seems essential across the discipline. Laudan, in contrast, allows for the possibility of different perspectives and objectives coexisting within a discipline and using the idea of Research Traditions as the means for differentiating the goals and work of subgroups of scientists. Toulmin's idea of goals derived through a process of "strategic consensus" seems appropriate to both philosophies with the major difference in the way the work of the discipline is divided (a single discipline versus multiple Research Traditions within one discipline). Laudan acknowledged that consensus on goals might not be possible and might not be necessary; his view of Research Traditions would allow for variation to exist within a single discipline. This view allows for greater variety and perhaps flexibility within a discipline while allowing for consistency within the discipline through the range of problems addressed within the field. Toulmin seems to share much of this perspective although giving greater emphasis to concepts as an important component in the continuity of the discipline over time.

Toulmin's emphasis on concepts is an obvious unique feature of his philosophy and warrants further consideration for its relevance to nursing. Although Laudan's philosophy is distinctive for giving weight to conceptual problems and elaborating on their importance within a scientific discipline, Toulmin (1972) places concepts at the center of the discussion of science. His ideas about concepts are reflected well in the statement that "every concept is an intellectual micro-institution" (p. 166). In Toulmin's view, concepts reflect not only the content of the current knowledge base of a discipline but also the techniques, symbolic representations, scope of application and ultimately scientists' judgments.

RELEVANCE FOR NURSING

Toulmin's approach to concepts presents some interesting contrasts with the large volume of nursing literature regarding theory development and the role of concepts in science. Concepts have been viewed as important components of knowledge development in nursing for some time (Chinn & Kramer, 1991; Walker & Avant, 1988, 1995) and numerous reports of analyses of concepts are available in the literature of nursing. Concepts are also discussed in the literature of other disciplines as critical components of knowledge development. In spite of the attention given to concepts, a thorough understanding of their nature and their role in knowledge development has not been evident in the literature of many disciplines (Rodgers, 2000a, 2000b).

Concepts typically have been viewed as names or symbols for aspects of observable reality as ideas or mental pictures or images or merely as words or parts of speech. The variety of discussions of concepts in the literature of nursing "raises questions about concepts in regard to processes of human thought, the relationship between concepts and empirical reality and between concepts and language, and the role of social contexts in concept development" (Rodgers, 2000b, pp. 10–11). Toulmin's work provides a detailed exploration of the potential contributions of concepts to understanding and the importance of their role in knowledge development. Building on this work contributes to a more thorough and philosophically substantive foundation for concept analysis work and expands the notion from that of merely "analysis" to the work of "concept development." Rodgers (2000a) has employed Toulmin's ideas in constructing an alternative approach to analysis of concepts, advocating, along with Toulmin, an emphasis on concept development as a fundamental activity of science.

For Toulmin, all scientific work is a process of concept development. His discussion of the content, organization, and conduct of science offers a unique way of envisioning the activities of scientists and for determining the rationality of scientific endeavors. The idea of science as a "scientific enterprise" gains a stronger foothold with Toulmin's position by showing not only the rules and structures involved but also providing some provocative ideas on the role of the scientists, the people at the center of all scientific effort, and the organizational structures that facilitate, deter, or otherwise serve to focus the work of science. Nursing can benefit from awareness of the various aspects of the context, both professional and social, that provide an ongoing structure and direction for knowledge development.

Toulmin's ideas of discipline and profession also provide significant insight in another area of nursing concern. The topic of whether or not nursing is a "discipline" has been prevalent throughout the recent history of nursing. Such discussion has included considerable argument and some confusion about whether nursing is a discipline, a profession or, perhaps the most popular alternative, a professional discipline. Distinctions between academic disciplines and professional disciplines have been proposed, which partially explains why nursing may function differently from other disciplines such as those in the more traditional sciences (sometimes referred to as the "hard" sciences). Physics and chemistry provide a useful comparison to illustrate this distinction. Toulmin's discussion of the matter might provide some useful insight into this debate for nursing. According to Toulmin's view, differences associated with a discipline such as nursing might be associated with contextual issues and the organization of the "profession" and not necessarily factors inherently associated with the discipline itself. For example, nurses work within a structure that is regulated by various laws and Practice Acts, which places significant boundaries around the scope of delivery of nursing care. While that situation gives feedback to the development of the discipline, it is not essential that the discipline itself be different from other academic entities. Nurses, therefore, can see their discipline and profession as having unique contextual factors that affect the profession component and not necessarily as having a disciplinary structure different from that of other disciplines.

Toulmin's view of science requires that a science have clear explanatory ideals. In the absence of those ideals, it is not possible to apply his formula to determine what problems exist that need to be addressed by further inquiry. This position is quite distinct from the views presented in other philosophies of science. The Logical Positivists, for example, do not address the goals of the science at all but look instead at the product (theory) produced and how it contributes to approximating Truth. Kuhn (1962/1970) sees science as the process of articulating a paradigm; for Laudan (1977), science takes place in accordance with specific research traditions in a discipline. The purposes and goals may only be implied in the case of paradigms and research traditions. Toulmin's approach, however, requires that the members of the discipline have a clear understanding of the discipline's overall focus and goals. Effort to delineate and gain agreement on goals can be very worthwhile in a discipline such as nursing that may seem disjointed at times due to its tremendous array of content and purposes. Toulmin's challenge was, in part, to demonstrate how a science maintains some consistency over time in addition to how change occurs in the conceptual repertoire. Attention to nursing's focus and goals and its conceptual transmit may reveal consistency in the work of nurse scholars throughout nursing's extensive history and provide focus for continuing progress.

CONCLUSION

Toulmin provides a unique entry in the area of Historicist views of science. One obvious innovation in his approach concerns his emphasis on concepts. Focusing on concepts to provide the core of a scientific field, Toulmin is able to describe the processes by which scientific change occurs, a primary emphasis in philosophy of science. Toulmin is also able, however, to capture elements of the process of science that account for continuity in a discipline over time, in other words, how disciplines maintain their core identify for an extended time. By focusing on concepts as a "transmit," he provides interesting elements about the social structure and processes of science and adds new dimensions and insights to historicist ideas of science. Toulmin, similar to Kuhn and Laudan, sees a significant role for people – the scientists – involved in the activity of science and expands the idea of science as an enterprise rather than as a specific type of knowledge. Through his work on concepts, the organization of disciplines, and the socialization of new scientists, Toulmin provides interesting ideas for consideration in the continuing growth and development of nursing knowledge. He maintains the seemingly practical nature of Laudan's emphasis on problem solving yet introduces social elements that help to explain how progress in resolving scientific problems can be evaluated. Toulmin's discussion of the ideals and the growth of intellectual disciplines also offers considerable insight for nurse scholars in the effort to understand the construction of nursing knowledge and the mechanisms of scientific change and progress in the discipline of nursing.

FOR DISCUSSION

1. For selected concepts of interest in nursing, discuss the concept's language, representation techniques, and scope of application.
2. Toulmin identifies a discipline as characterized by explanatory goals, a repertory of concepts and procedures, and the accumulated experience of scientists. Discuss how this characterization fits with nursing as a discipline.

3. Compare the status of nursing as a discipline to Toulmin's ideas of compact, diffuse, and would-be disciplines.

4. Discuss Forums of Competition as they might operate in the context of nursing for the development of concepts.

5. Discuss ways in which new scientists are enculturated in regard to nursing's conceptual transmit.

REFERENCES

Chinn, P. L., & Kramer, M. (1991). *Theory and nursing: A systematic approach* (3rd ed.). St. Louis: C. V. Mosby.

Darwin, C. (1859). *On the origin of species by means of natural selection or the preservation of favoured races in the struggle for life.* London: J. Murray

Feyerabend, P. (1975). *Against method.* London: Verso.

Kuhn, T. S. (1957). *The Copernican revolution: Planetary astronomy in the development of Western thought.* Cambridge: Harvard University Press.

Kuhn, T. S. (1970). *The structure of scientific revolutions* (2nd ed.). Chicago: University of Chicago. (originally published 1962).

Laudan, L. (1977). *Progress and its problems.* Berkeley: University of California Press.

Reichenbach, H. (1938). *Experience and prediction: An analysis of the foundations and the structure of knowledge.* Chicago: University of Chicago Press.

Rodgers, B. L. (2000a). Concept analysis: An evolutionary view. In B. L. Rodgers and K. A. Knafl (Eds.), *Concept development in nursing: Foundations, techniques, and applications* (2nd ed.) (pp. 77–102). Philadelphia: W. B. Saunders.

Rodgers, B. L. (2000b). Philosophical foundations of concept development. In B. L. Rodgers and K. A. Knafl (Eds.), *Concept development in nursing: Foundations, techniques, and applications* (2nd ed.). (pp. 7–38). Philadelphia: W. B. Saunders.

Toulmin, S. (1953). *The philosophy of science: An introduction.* London: Hutchinson's University Library.

Toulmin, S. (1972). *Human understanding.* Princeton, NJ: Princeton University Press.

Walker, L. O., & Avant, K. C. (1988). *Strategies for theory construction in nursing* (2nd ed.). Norwalk, CT: Appleton & Lange.

Walker, L. O., & Avant, K. C. (1995). *Strategies for theory construction in nursing* (3rd ed.). Norwalk, CT: Appleton & Lange.

CHAPTER 9

The Postmodern Turn

KEY IDEAS

deconstruction	postmodernism
discourse	poststructuralism
margins	power
metanarrative	praxis
narrative knowledge	structuralism

The Historicist period signaled a major transition from the rigidity of Logical Positivism to a view of science that incorporates values, context, and the human element in science. Although it might be tempting to say that Logical Positivism no longer exists at least as a philosophical movement, it would be shortsighted to attribute that status to any philosophical tradition. As in nursing or any field for that matter, each wave of thought in philosophy will have evolved from what existed previously. In that sense, philosophies never really die and everything is "post" something.

POSTMODERNISM

The first challenge—and an enduring one—to understanding what is referred to as **postmodernism** in philosophy is securing a definition of this tradition. This is a nearly impossible task because the very essence of postmodernism would seem to eschew a single definition. Instead, as was the case with the traditions discussed previously, there are examples and variants that can be explored to provide insight into the multitude of ways in which postmodernism appears in philosophy.

In an introduction to postmodernism, Cahoone (1996) captures the confusion and highly-charged nature of the term "postmodernism" in his historical overview of the development of this tradition. Citing the increasing popularity of the postmodern "label," he points out that

> Philosophical opinion regarding the postmodern family is deeply divided. For some, postmodernism connotes the final escape from the stultifying legacy of modern European theology, metaphysics, authoritarianism, colonialism, racism, and domination. To others it represents the attempt by disgruntled left-wing intellectuals to destroy Western civilization. To yet others it labels a goofy collection of hermetically obscure writers who are really talking about nothing at all. (p. 1)

Referring to all these reactions as "misguided," Cahoone points out that it is a "mistake to seek a single, essential meaning applicable to all the term's instances" (p. 1). Instead the distinguishing features of postmodernism are more easily identified through recognition of a common, broad ontology or "world-view" and value statements regarding the origins of knowledge and its role in contemporary societies.

Basic Tenet of Postmodernism

There is, therefore, no single definition of postmodernism that can convey its meaning and intent. However, one tenet of postmodernism characterizes the domain of the ideology. The statement "the center does not hold" might be considered the rallying cry of postmodernists and appears in numerous writings about the postmodern period along with associated philosophy.[1] The statement, adapted from "The Second Coming" by the poet William Butler Yeats, appears in the following excerpt:

> Turning and turning in the widening gyre
> The falcon cannot hear the falconer;
> Things fall apart; the centre cannot hold;
> Mere anarchy is loosed upon the world,
> The blood-dimmed tide is loosed, and everywhere
> The ceremony of innocence is drowned;
> The best lack all conviction, while the worst
> Are full of passionate intensity. (Yeats, 1976)[2]

---

[1]See, for example, articles by Marshall (2000), Lim (2000), and Tiemann (1993).
[2]Original publication c. 1918.

In this poem Yeats continues to describe a second coming and a beastly figure emerging into his sight. Yeats presents a rather apocalyptic view in this poem and there has been considerable debate about this poem's elements and their reference to specific persons, ideologies, and events. The similarities that exist with the idea of the center giving way have caused this expression to appear in discussions of postmodern ideology.

The modern period of philosophy was characterized, to a great extent, by a belief in universals, absolutes, and Truth. Prevailing thought advocated for a single reality that served as a foundation against which all knowledge could be evaluated and determined to be True or not-True. The Positivists believed particularly in the power of science, which they defined as being consistent with strict empiricism, to achieve knowledge that was infallible and corresponded with that singular reality.

For the Postmodernists, that foundation—a belief in a single reality that provided a unifying and stable center—is discarded. It is not discarded because of mere dislike or preference, however, but because it is considered indefensible. The idea of a center promotes uniformity and oppression and fails to recognize the value and, in fact, the reality that individuals inhabit multiple worlds and have multiple realms and differing perspectives of their experiences. In other words, people are believed to construct their own realities and those constructions must be recognized, valued, brought to the forefront, or "given voice" in any human inquiry.

Postmodernism is a rejection of what sometimes are called master narratives or **metanarratives** (Lyotard, 1984, p. xxiv), which present singular answers and descriptions presumed to fit the lives, experiences, and meanings of all human beings (see Box 9-1). It is, in this regard, a curious blend of science, culture, behavior, politics, and literature. The scientific element is derived from the application of methodology to gain understanding. The tie to culture is reflected in the indi-

BOX 9-1

POSTMODERNISM

Postmodernism presents the rejection of "metanarratives" or single descriptions of reality that are presumed to be applicable to all people and situations. Instead multiple truths and realities are recognized, and power relationships that exist in the sharing of knowledge must be acknowledged as important in all knowledge claims.

Postmodernism acknowledges the effect of social, cultural, economic, and other factors in claims about knowledge. Multiple interpretations are possible for all events, and the focus of investigation often is to identify the less obvious meanings and messages said to occupy the "margins."

vidual constructions people create for their worlds which to a great extent are derived from social and cultural influences.

Role of Discourse

The postmodern link to literature and literary ideas is a particularly interesting one with relevance for nursing. The term "discourse" is featured prominently in much of the literature of postmodernism. **Discourse**, in the postmodern tradition, refers to the pivotal role of language in human existence. Language carries with it diverse social, political, and cultural meanings that reflect the group's status and values and also help to shape that group as its members and as the group as a whole develop. This language can be examined to reveal both the overt and the more subtle messages in the language exchange. In fact, discourse analysis is a popular form of inquiry among literary critics and some of the seminal work on discourse comes from the field of literary criticism and rhetoric. Discourse, however, also captures the ways in which medical and health phenomena are conveyed in the literature and the relationships among care providers and care recipients when they are discussing health situations. The language chosen to convey ideas is more than mere words but presents underlying value statements in addition to informational content. As an example, consider the recent change from the phrase "sexually transmitted disease" to "sexually transmitted infection" in an attempt to avoid the affront associated with identifying someone as having a "disease" and to convey a less stigmatizing image of a hopefully treatable "infection."

Discourse goes beyond language, however, to include human beings' actions and behaviors. A statement is not merely a combination of words; it is an interaction between the speaker and the listener, or the originator of the speech and the recipient. Nonverbal human interactions work the same way in that actions and behaviors send messages subject to interpretation and response. Human words, other forms of communication, and behavior are all subject to analysis as forms of discourse.

To a great extent, Postmodernism is a reaction to the industrialization of society, the emergence (and potential dominance) of technology, and the continuing reliance on an elevated status (or super-legitimation) of "science." The French philosopher Jean-François Lyotard argued that science itself constitutes a form of discourse (p. 3), and the transformations that have occurred in modern societies of the 20th century "have altered the game rules for science, literature, and the arts" (Lyotard, 1984, p. xxiii). He continued, stating that

> science has always been in conflict with narratives...to the extent that science does not restrict itself to stating useful regularities and seeks the truth, it is obliged to legitimate the rules of its own game. It then produces a discourse of legitimation with respect to its own status, a discourse called philosophy. (p. xxiii)

Lyotard viewed science as a self-legitimizing approach to knowledge that presented its own kind of "discourse" (p. 3). It had been considered an exteriorized form of knowledge, devoid of any intrinsic involvement of the person doing the "knowing." It was thought to be a product of rigorous research not something constructed by human beings, the scientists. With the postmodern shift, however, science could no longer be viewed as an end itself or as a product to be valued for its own sake but as a produced and exchanged commodity that had value primarily in its commodified form (pp. 4–5). Lyotard (1984) encouraged recognition of the value-commodity status of science in addition to acknowledging that "scientific knowledge does not represent the totality of knowledge: it has always existed in addition to, and in competition and conflict with, another kind of knowledge," which Lyotard referred to as **"narrative knowledge"** (p. 7).

STRUCTURALISM

The application of scientific principles to the study of society had led to the emergence of a theoretical tradition known as **structuralism**, developed in its early forms by Swiss linguist Ferdinand de Saussure (1959) and promoted by anthropologist Claude Levi-Strauss (1963). The structuralism of Levi-Strauss placed a primary emphasis on the overriding structures that influence human and group behavior. Structures that affect people include language, relationships, traditions and rituals, etc., which influence the development of the self as well as the social group. This approach to the study of human beings as existing in structured societies is in stark contrast to the strong emphasis that earlier philosophers, such as Marx, the phenomenologists, and psychoanalytic theorists, placed on the *self* (Cahoone, 1996). In a way, structuralism was an attempt to apply scientific principles to the study of societies and cultures, that is, looking for rules and causal relationships to explain societies and social behavior that are wholly human constructions. This structuralist approach recognized the role of culture and other human elements in constructing realities and rejected the reduction of human nature to more traditional scientific phenomena. It did seek, however, to maintain the air of rigor and objectivity appropriate to a "scientific" study of humankind.

POSTSTRUCTURALISM

The poststructuralists, such as Gilles Deleuze (1983, 1993), Jacques Derrida (1974), and Michel Foucault (1972a, 1972b, 1977), accepted the ideology of socially constructed realities but differed from a structuralist approach in that they rejected any semblance of science. Their approach instead was to focus the techniques of inquiry on an examination of the cultures themselves particularly as culture was enmeshed in literature and other human creations. The examination of these human constructions was expected to provide insight into the way in which cultures influenced the realities and the messages and meanings contained within the media of language and other cultural relics.

Rather than describing how to build knowledge, postmodernism and **poststructuralism** pose a direct challenge to the dominant ideas of unity, oneness, uniformity, Truth, and foundationalism. A positive contribution comes in the method of inquiry offered by the philosophers of this genre and the techniques they created for reflexively exploring the ways in which meanings have been constructed and conveyed. A post-structuralist approach to inquiry is essentially the deconstruction of what exists. Rather than examining situations particularly language and practices, the task of poststructuralist inquiry is to deconstruct the text to identify the disputable messages and influences as if they possess absolute or immutable meanings.

Derrida (1974), one of the most notable of the poststructuralists, refers to this shift in perspective as "the end of the book and the beginning of writing." Derrida transfers the focus of analysis from finished objects to the act of creating the objects. In his seminal work, *Of Grammatology*, he explains the movement away from speech as the most important form of language. Previously in linguistics, speech had held the highest regard because of the "presence" of the speaker; the speaker must be in the situation for speech to occur. Writing, in contrast, had been regarded merely as the transcription of speech. Although this is an instrumental function of language, it gives writing a lower status than speech due to the absent speaker in written forms of communication. Derrida (1974) foretold the "death of speech," meaning essentially that it had been subordinated and no longer maintained a privileged position in language. Similarly the idea of writing comes to mean more than the simple act of placing words (or speech) on paper, the instrumental function of writing, as noted previously. In this sense, writing includes film, dance, and other fine and performing arts. Derrida removes the speaker from the center of the processes of speaking and writing and emphasizes the reader who consumes or interprets the text.

Deconstruction

Shifting emphasis to the reader rather than maintaining focus on the speaker reveals that multiple interpretations are possible for any text. Rather than only one valid meaning for a speech act or section of text, there are many ways of interpreting or understanding what is there to read or hear. Meaning and interpretations can be revealed through a process of deconstruction, showing the contradictions that exist in the work and the many possible messages being conveyed. **Deconstruction** strives to "locate the promising marginal text" (Derrida, 1974, p. xvii), or the hidden or less obvious messages that are present. According to Derrida (1974), certain terms hold a "resident hierarchy" (p. xxvii), a situation nurse theorist Jean Watson (1999) relates to the privileged status of "medicine" and "cure" in western health care systems. "Nursing" and "care" which, according to Watson, represent subordinate ideas, occupy a background position, or a position Derrida would refer to as being in the **margins**. In other words, the focus on medicine and cure in much of health literature pushes aside the polar ideas of nursing and care; because of their absence from discussion, they take on a "marginal" position.

The process of deconstruction strives to reverse the "resident hierarchy" by revealing the marginalized terminology and ideas and to reconstruct the text in a way that gives foreground status to ideas previously commanded to the background (or margin). By doing so, meanings hidden but still highly influential in their subtlety or complete absence are revealed along with the cultural values embedded in the text. Such awareness and deconstruction make evident the ways in which presumed truths, such as the emphasis on "cure," actually are socially constructed and result from prevailing values and emphasis in society.

FOUCAULT'S APPLICATIONS TO HISTORY

The French philosopher, Foucault, demonstrates the application of some of these ideas to the understanding of history. In *The Archaeology of Knowledge*, Foucault (1972a) describes the tradition in historical inquiry of seeking long periods of stability and linkages among seemingly disparate events (p. 3). Historians have focused on relationships and continuities, assuming that the series of events was known, and "it was simply a question of defining the position of each element in relation to the other elements in the series" (p. 7). For Foucault, however, the focus needed to be on identifying the series, determining its nature and associated events, and addressing the changes and transformations that occurred. According to Foucault, the process of history formerly was to "memorize the *monuments* of the past, transform them into *documents*, and lend speech to these traces which, in themselves, are often not verbal, or which say in silence something other than what they actually say; in our time, history transforms *documents* into *monuments*" (p. 7). Here Foucault advocates against the usual practice of historians of constructing a "total history" (p. 9), a sort of grand description of a time or period. Such total history is seen in how time periods are identified in broad terms such as the Byzantine era or Colonial America. Such notation gives the impression that there are structured, delimitable, and identifiable times or events in the history of civilization. Foucault argues that there should be a shift toward a "general history," which reveals that many different possible configurations of a period exist on many different levels.

This idea of history as involving multiple ways of configuring events and connections and particularly of examining discontinuity and transformations is consistent with Foucault's notion of knowledge and power. **Power**, according to Foucault, is not the possession of an individual or a group but is more widely dispersed and operates in a variety of relationships and interchanges. Typically people are not aware of its operations; this lack of awareness actually is critical to the continuance of the power relationship. It is easy to see how once a person recognizes that another has "power," the nature of the relationship immediately can shift. Consequently lack of awareness keeps the power relationship as it is. Knowledge is a significant purveyor of power, and the two are so closely linked that Foucault uses the term power/knowledge to reflect the connection among these two elements. Power/knowledge promotes and limits behaviors, rewarding individuals who act in a manner consistent with desired behaviors.

The connection of these ideas with the literary turn of Derrida and others can now be seen: Language is an important medium for power/knowledge. Discursive practices (speech acts) reveal existing power/knowledge systems. As such, they are important subjects for analysis not because they possess any discernible truth value but because it is important to understand their origin and history and the way in which *claims* about truth reveal power relationships.

Foucault's position on truth as embodying a tremendous amount of social value and power is evident in the following passage where he describes five important characteristics of truth:

> [Truth] is centered on the form of scientific discourse and the institutions which produce it; it is subject to constant economic and political incitement (the demand for truth, as much for economic production as for political power); it is the object, under diverse forms, of immense diffusion and consumption (circulating through apparatuses of education and information whose extent is relatively broad in the social body, not withstanding certain strict limitations); it is produced and transmitted under the control, dominant if not exclusive, of a few great political and economic apparatuses (university, Army, writing, media); lastly it is the issue of a whole political debate and social confrontation ('ideological') struggles. (Foucault, 1972b, pp. 131–132)

Describing truth (or knowledge) as inherently associated with power, Foucault argues that the challenge is not merely to free truth from the entrapment of systems of power. Such an accomplishment would not be possible because, after all, truth *is* power. Instead the need is for "detaching the power of truth from the forms of hegemony, social, economic, and cultural, within which it operates at the present time" (Foucault, 1972b, p. 133).

Writers of the poststructuralist genre reject the phenomenologists' idea that a person has a subjective identity or essence. Instead he or she has varying ways of revealing the self, as a discourse about the self. The sense of self or individual identity is evident to others through actions, behaviors, and other forms of communication (Cahoone, 1996; Derrida, 1974; Foucault, 1972a, 1972b). Poststructuralist inquiry is focused on language specifically the discourse that exists and the power relationships it reveals. Poststructuralist analysis seeks to identify the power relationships revealed through forms of discourse. In a manner consistent with the ideology of deconstruction, it is often as important to reveal what *is not* said as it is to notice what is said.

APPLICATIONS OF POSTMODERNISM IN NURSING

Poststructuralist Inquiry

Postmodern approaches to inquiry can provide valuable insight into a wide variety of phenomena and situations of interest to nurses (see Box 9-2). For example, mental health constitutes one area in which poststructuralist inquiry has been applied in nursing. Dzurec (1995) provides an historical account of "mental disability" and the ways in which treatment approaches often fail people affected by mental health concerns. Through her argument, she associated treatment failures with "unspoken values that pervade American life and constitute profoundly visible yet hidden assumptions that drive thinking and action concerning severe mental disability" (p. 251). Some of these values are reflected in the preference for "work over welfare, upward over downward mobility, high over low status, independence over dependence," and other values, as well as assumptions about the scarcity of resources available to treat various conditions (p. 251). Dzurec demonstrates the value of using alternate perspectives to examine an accepted situation and gain new forms of understanding (Dzurec, 1989).

Deconstruction

Poststructuralist approaches have been applied to other areas of concern in nursing. Rodgers (1991) used a process of deconstruction to explore the origins and implications of prevailing dogma in nursing. Common propositions about nursing were examined to demonstrate the context and incentives for the emergence of accepted ideology in nursing. Nursing has been described, for example, as "an art and a science," and as a "professional discipline," in contrast to an academic discipline. Other statements, such as those regarding the nature of human beings or the role of nurses interacting with human beings, convey a considerable amount of information about perceptions and values in addition to the content immediately apparent on reading a statement. Phillips (1993) also applied techniques of

---

BOX 9-2

POSTMODERN INQUIRY

Postmodern Inquiry includes
    Poststructuralist analysis
    Deconstruction
    Discourse analysis

    Narrative analysis
    Feminist analysis

deconstruction to an understanding of "caring" and argued that the continued emphasis on caring as nearly synonymous with nursing puts an undue emphasis on emotional aspects of care.

Such techniques also can be applied to common health care situations and popular media. A recent review of several publications targeted for readers who are HIV positive revealed numerous ads depicting people engaging in athletic activities, smiling and holding a single pill, proclaiming one pill a day is all that is needed for continued health and well-being for people with positive HIV status. While incredible strides have been made in the treatment of HIV, the messages sent by such ads also may have unintended consequences such as minimizing the importance of self care, prevention, and following available treatment regimens.

As another example, consider the idea of certain types of research as "hard," and others as "soft." The use of these terms alone conveys images of rigor and soundness or the lack thereof in certain methods for research. Aspects of science intended to explain and "control" are sometimes said to convey a patriarchal view of nature as something to be dominated. A poststructuralist approach to inquiry sees research, instead, as "an enactment of power relations; the focus is on the development of a mutual dialogic production of a multi-voice, multi-centered discourse" (Lather, 1991, p. 112). In a manner characteristic of the postmodern movement, Lather calls for a rejection of the preoccupation with objectivity and, in its place, attention to questions of race, class, gender, power, motivation, and authority in all inquiry (p. 113). According to the poststructuralist tradition, researchers need to consider their own biases and preconceptions that shape even the first ideas associated with the inquiry. In other words, the initial recognition and labeling of some situation as a problem for study reflects the investigator's perspective. A study of resilience, for example, may imply or may reveal the reseacher's hidden notions that some people have unexpected strengths or resources not considered characteristic of members of a particular group. Without an expectation of being downtrodden in the face of adversity, would concepts such as resilience exist or would their forms and content be different?

Such observations and types of inquiry reveal what may be unintended outcomes of discourse or they may be subtle ways of reinforcing specific ideology about the situations being presented. According to those advocating a postmodern approach, recognition of the power inherent in all discourse is important to advancing a more complete understanding of human experience. Postmodernism compels researchers to consider just such questions as they embark on their inquiry. The same reflexivity is warranted even in everyday conversation, or teaching, or writing. Language conveys all sorts of messages and meanings; the way in which situations are framed carries a variety of judgments and preconceptions. For nurses, language provides a foundation that allows the uniqueness of each individual to emerge rather than forcing stereotypes or conformity with generalizations. It is helpful to remember the slogan of the postmodern movement that "the center does not hold" (adapted from Yeats, 1976). Each person instead becomes his or her own center and multiple realities are supported and encouraged.

Employing Plurality in Research

For nursing research, one of the most striking outcomes of the shift to postmodernism is a greatly expanded array of methodologies to use in inquiry. Numerous authors in nursing have advocated "pluralism" or a multiplistic approach to research (Coward, 1990; Letourneau & Allen, 1999; Phillips, 2001). With the demise of a belief in Absolute Truth and continued debate about the value and nature of objectivity as a proper concern in research, methodologies have been developed that capitalize on the subjective nature of experience. Qualitative research in general has experienced a tremendous increase in popularity and methodologic development since the 1970s when postmodern ideas began to garner attention.[1] Researchers in nursing and in other disciplines use methods consistent with postmodern ideology with increasing frequency to capture the unique realities of individuals. It is important to recognize that researchers using quantitative methods also may view their results as only partial views of reality rather than advocating the broad and sweeping generalizations more common in earlier scientific periods, particularly those aligned with Logical Positivism. New methodologies also have emerged; they are referred to as narrative inquiry, discourse analysis, feminist research, and post-structuralist inquiry (Carr, 1996; Hallett, Austin, & Luker, 2000; Jorgensen & Phillips, 2002; Naples, 2003; Phillips, 2002; Powers, 1996; Traynor, 1996; Weiss & Wodak, 2003).

Praxis

The term "**praxis**," which has become increasingly commonplace as a part of this movement, is used to capture the integration of formerly disparate realms of subjective and objective existence (Thorne & Hayes, 1996). The term, which is quite common in some literature, is used as a substitute for "practice" or even "action." Although definitions of praxis are infrequent in the literature, the common use reveals its reference to behavior or action based on knowledge and values. It is not merely "doing" but doing in a way that reflects the total being, or who one *is* as a person. The notion of "praxis" captures the idea that the ways in which nurses (or any people) behave and interact is a result of not just knowing what to do but also a reflection of the philosophical assumptions and the socialization of the person.

Postmodernism challenges longstanding perspectives on the nature of knowledge and encourages new approaches to understanding the world and especially the humans who inhabit it. It is a philosophy that would seem immediately com-

---

[1]It is important to recognize that not all qualitative research fits the postmodern tradition. While attention to language, discourse, and narrative are consistent with postmodernism, thus the idea of narrative- or interview-based data gained a foothold, it is possible to do "empirical" qualitative research. A researcher may do qualitative research yet still believe in the idea of Truth. Clearly there is a strong connection between methods and philosophy, yet even this is not absolute.

fortable to nurses, who are accustomed to listening to and valuing uniqueness and individuality. It also challenges nurses to seek other forms of knowledge beyond the narrow conceptions of "science." In fact, some authors justify the divergent approaches to knowledge development, which create an imposing contrast with science, by pointing out that the study of human beings constitutes a unique realm, that of the *human sciences*. These human sciences pose a contrast with the natural sciences, require unique modes of investigation, and of course carry different criteria for credibility.

In addition to these effects of the postmodern turn in philosophy and a corresponding influence on the development of knowledge, there can be a broader impact on nursing practice and the organization and delivery of nursing services. Watson (1999) describes the postmodern era in regard to the "erosion" of Western culture (p. 47). Postmodernism challenges the stereotypes and hierarchies that have been embedded in, for example, the dominance of medicine over nursing, masculine over feminine, and science over other forms of knowledge. Taking advantage of the opportunities presented by such philosophical thought—indeed postmodernism is essentially a cultural change not merely a different form of epistemology—requires that nursing, "poised between two worlds and times" (Watson, 1999, p. 47), reconsider its roles and identity, and "face some new truths about its power and possibilities" (Watson, 1999, p. 47). The opportunity exists for the emergence of a care, rather than a cure, mentality and for revisions in the definition of nursing and its knowledge base.

CONCLUSION

There can be no question that postmodernism provokes considerable reflection on tradition and what has been accepted as "truth." However, every philosophical viewpoint has significant limitations or at least questions that require further consideration before adopting a position. Postmodernism casts doubt on some prevailing notions of knowledge and science. In a sense, it pulls the foundation out from under most of what researchers might believe about building a knowledge base (arguing, for example, that knowledge is constructed rather than discovered). In the support of pluralism in the approach to knowledge, postmodernism offers little insight into how to evaluate the quality of knowledge, or which knowledge claims might be more warranted than others. It creates a truth by argument rather than by evidence approach or at least allows for alternate forms of evidence to prevail beyond the usual sensory data. These characteristics are some of the major strengths of postmodernism yet they represent some areas of greatest concern. Even if scientists accept that knowledge has the potential to reflect various biases, the question remains whether biases should be acknowledged or if it is more appropriate to attempt to control them (even if complete objectivity is not possible). In the postmodern tradition, some argument exists that one set of biases can best be counteracted by invoking another opposing set of biases (see especially Feminism, Chapter 11).

As with any philosophical position, careful scrutiny is appropriate to ensure that both claims to knowledge and claims about the nature of inquiry are defensible and sound. On one level, the postmodern era and associated developments in philosophy support the creativity and innovativeness that philosopher Paul Feyerabend (1975) claimed were so lacking in more traditional approaches when he called for an "anything goes" approach to inquiry. Scholars recognize, of course, that in real life not everything is acceptable; all alternatives do not work to the same degree. Inquiry consistent with the principles of postmodernism continues on philosophical and methodological levels. Nurses can be and have been important contributors to the continuing development and refinement of this line of thought, helping to shape this emerging tradition.

 ## FOR DISCUSSION

1. Compare and contrast the Postmodern tradition with the major tenets of Logical Positivism and Historicism.
2. For a particular phenomenon or concept, discuss the ways in which social, economic, education, culture, and individual values can influence how the phenomenon is viewed.
3. Discuss the meanings and messages conveyed in a current health related news report or advertisement.
4. Discuss implications for nursing knowledge development associated with the idea of science as a "commodity."
5. Discuss criteria for evaluating the value and usefulness of research based on postmodern philosophy.

REFERENCES

Cahoone, L. (1996). Introduction. In L. Cahoone (Ed.), *Modernism to postmodernism: An anthology* (pp. 1–23). Cambridge, MA: Blackwell Publishers.

Carr, G. (1996). Themes relating to sexuality that emerged from a discourse analysis of the *Nursing Times* during 1980–1990. *Journal of Advanced Nursing, 24*, 196–212.

Coward, D. D. (1990). Critical multiplism: A research strategy for nursing science. *Image: Journal of Nursing Scholarship, 22*, 163–167.

Deleuze, G. (1983). *Nietzsche and philosophy* (H. Tomlinson, Trans.). New York: Columbia University Press.

Deleuze, G. (1993). *The Deleuze reader* (C. V. Boundas, Ed). New York: Columbia University Press.

Derrida, J. (1974). *Of grammatology* (G. C. Spivak, Trans.). Baltimore: Johns Hopkins University Press.

Dzurec, L. C. (1989). The necessity and evolution of multiple paradigms for nursing research: A poststructuralist perspective. *Advances in Nursing Science, 11*(4), 69–79.

Dzurec, L. C. (1995). Severe mental disability? Or a play of wills? In A. Omery, C. E. Kasper, & G. G. Page (Eds.), *In search of nursing science* (pp. 245–260). Thousand Oaks, CA: Sage Publications.

Feyerabend, P. (1975). *Against method*. London: Verso.

Foucault, M. (1972a). *The archaeology of knowledge* (A. M. S. Smith, Trans.). New York: Pantheon Books.

Foucault, M. (1972b). Truth and power, interview by A. Fontana and P. Pasquino (C. Gordin, Trans.), *Power/Knowledge: Selected interviews and other writings 1972–1977*. NY: Pantheon Books.

Foucault, M. (1977). Nietzsche, genealogy, history (D. B. S. Simon, Trans.). In D. Bouchard (Ed.), *Language, counter-memory, practise* (pp. 139–164). Ithaca, NY: Cornell University Press.

Hallett, C. E., Austin, L., & Luker, K. A. (2000). Community nurses' perceptions of patient 'compliance' in wound care: A discourse analysis. *Journal of Advanced Nursing, 32*(1), 115–123.

Jorgensen, M., & Phillips, L. (2002). *Discourse analysis as theory and method*. Thousand Oaks, CA: Sage Publications.

Lather, P. (1991). *Getting smart: Feminist research and pedagogy with/in the postmodern*. New York: Routledge.

Letourneau, N., & Allen, M. (1999). Post-positivistic critical multiplism: A beginning dialogue. *Journal of Advanced Nursing, 30*, 623–630.

Levi-Strauss, C. (1963). *Structural anthropology* (C. Jacobson, & B. G. Schoepf, Trans.). New York: Basic Books.

Lim, S. G. (2000). The center can(not) hold: American studies and global feminism. *American Studies International, 38*(3), 25–35.

Lyotard, J. F. (1984). *The postmodern condition: A report on knowledge* (G. B. B. Massumi, Trans.). Minneapolis, MN: University of Minnesota Press. (Original work published 1979)

Marshall, J. M. (November 20, 2000). Does the center hold? *The American Prospect, 11*(24), 14.

Naples, N. A. (2003). *Feminism and method: Ethnography, discourse analysis, and activist research*. New York: Routledge.

Phillips, D. A. (2001). Methodology for social accountability: Multiple methods and feminist, poststructural, psychoanalytic discourse analysis. *Advances in Nursing Science, 23*, 49–66.

Phillips, N. H., & Hardy, C. (2002). *Discourse analysis: Investigating processes of social construction*. Thousand Oaks, CA: Sage Publications.

Phillips, P. (1993). A deconstruction of caring. *Journal of Advanced Nursing, 18*, 1554–1558.

Powers, P. (1996). Discourse analysis as a methodology for nursing inquiry. *Nurs Inq 1996 Dec; 3*(4):207–17.

Rodgers, B. L. (1991). Deconstructing the dogma in nursing knowledge and practice. *Image: Journal of Nursing Scholarship, 23*, 177–181.

Saussure, F. de (1959). *Course in general linguistics* (W. Baskin, Trans.). New York: Philosophical Library.

Thorne, S. E., & Hayes, V. E. (Eds.). (1996). *Nursing praxis: Knowledge and action*. Thousand Oaks, CA: Sage Publications.

Tiemann, K. A. (1993) On making the center hold. *Teaching Sociology, 21*, 257–258.

Traynor, M. (1996). Looking at discourse in a literature review of nursing texts. *Journal of Advanced Nursing, 23*, 1155–1161.

Watson, J. (1999). *Postmodern nursing and beyond*. Edinburgh: Churchill Livingstone.

Weiss, G., & Wodak, R. (Eds.). (2003). *Critical discourse analysis: Theory and interdisciplinarity*. New York: Palgrave Macmillan.

Yeats, W. B. (1976). The second coming. In F. Tuohy, *Yeats* (p. 168). New York: Macmillan.

CHAPTER 10

Interpretive Inquiry: The Mirror Cracked[1]

KEY IDEAS

action	hermeneutics
communicative action	interpretations
Critical Social Theory	linguisticality
Dasein	praxis
Frankfurt School	preunderstanding
fusion of horizons	speech
hermeneutic circle	text

The rise of postmodernism in philosophy brought about a number of new traditions of inquiry. The prominence of narrative and the possibility of deconstruction (Derrida, 1974; Mueller-Vollmer, 1988) were just two developments associated with this movement. Poststructuralist ideology also accompanied the beginning of the postmodern movement, a turn away from the application of "scientific" principles to the study of human beings and their social organization. In

---

[1]The reference is to a 1980 movie based on Agatha Christie's (1962) novel, *The Mirror Crack'd from Side to Side*. The reference to a mirror is derived from the philosophical idea of the mind as a mirror, related to correspondence theories of truth. See also Rorty (1979), *Philosophy and the Mirror of Nature*. The fact that this title is drawn from a mystery novel is not accidental.

general, postmodernism (as discussed in Chapter 9) calls for a turn away from the idea of absolute objectivity and at minimum a pluralistic approach to inquiry. In this contemporary view, it is essential to recognize people's unique realities and multiple truths as individuals and as members of groups and cultures.

Two other forms of inquiry also gained prominence as part of the postmodern shift. To some extent, Hermeneutics reflects the linguistics focus present in Derrida's writing. Critical Social Theory, another prominent ideology, reflects the idea of power hierarchies that was such a prominent component of poststructuralism particularly from the perspective of Foucault. These traditions are consistent with recent developments in philosophy and are the appropriate next step in an examination of newer movements in philosophy as well as implications for nursing inquiry. These two philosophical traditions are quite different when compared to each other; they will be discussed separately in this chapter. They have much in common, however, due to their positions in the overall genre of postmodern ideology.

 ## THE HERMENEUTIC TRADITION

Although **Hermeneutics** appears to be a relatively recent development in philosophy due to its resurgence as a method of inquiry around the 1980s, this philosophy has a very long history that dates to the 1600s and likely earlier. The philosophy actually may be derived from Aristotle's work on rhetoric. Despite this long history, Hermeneutics received little attention in the literature of any of the "sciences" until fairly recently when it reappeared along with the similar ideologies associated with postmodernism. It is not a new tradition in practice, having been applied for centuries as a form of literary exegesis. However, the emergence of Hermeneutics in philosophy and its acceptance as a distinct form of inquiry with relevance for research are postmodern developments.

The term "hermeneutics" is derived rather indirectly from the name of the Greek messenger God, Hermes. The name Hermes gave rise to the Greek terms *hermēneutikos,* which is derived from *hermēneutēs,* which means "interpreter," and from *hermēneuein,* "to interpret." German derivatives include the terms *hermmēneuein,* which means "to interpret" and *hermēneutike* as the "art of interpretation" (Honderich, 1995). According to mythology, Hermes' role was to deliver messages from the gods to the common people. Performing that role required that Hermes be able to bridge the gap of understanding between the gods and the people; in other words, he had to be able to speak the languages of both (Mueller-Vollmer, 1988). Hermes' role and capability provide general insight into the nature of Hermeneutics as the act or process of interpretation. In the tradition of Hans-Georg Gadamer (1975, 1976), one of the most prominent figures in current discussions of hermeneutics, hermeneutics is a process of bridging the gaps that exist in attempts among humans to arrive at understanding.

In its most general form, Hermeneutics is a process of **interpretation** sometimes referred to as the art of interpretation (Mueller-Vollmer, 1988). In some of its earliest use, Hermeneutics was applied to the exploration of religious texts in an attempt to understand the basic meaning and intent of Holy Scriptures. Such inquiry was attempted to provide clarity regarding text content and avoid the church's apparent need to impose its own interpretation. From its earliest development, Hermeneutics has gone through considerable evolution as a process of interpretation particularly during the 19th and 20th centuries. Friedrich Schleiermacher (Redeker, 1973), one of the primary forces in the more recent development of Hermeneutics, emphasized the linguistic aspects of understanding and helped to position Hermeneutics as a scholarly endeavor. Other prominent individuals in the development of Hermeneneutics include the historians Wilhelm von Humboldt (1963) and Johann Gustav Droysen (1977), and philosophers Immanuel Kant (1965), Wilhelm Dilthey (1976), Ernst Cassirer (1944), and Edmund Husserl (1970). More recently, the German philosopher Gadamer (1975) has occupied a critical role, as have Jürgen Habermas (1971, 1984) and Martin Heidegger (1962, 1971).

In spite of the variations in specific approaches, there is considerable common ground among views classified as hermeneutic. In general, the problem of Hermeneutics is to bring what is unfamiliar into understanding. This goal is most clear when contrasted with the usual goal of epistemology, which is "to know," or of traditional science, which has the goal to develop theory, achieve greater probability, and determine cause and effect relationships. Hermeneutics, instead, has as its goal "understanding" or "enlightenment"—that is, the ability to say "I understand." Understanding involves the integration of information into present ways of seeing. It is a process of fully recognizing the speaker's or writer's message not merely hearing or seeing its varied fragments. When a person understands, he or she is changed in some way because the person incorporates newly discovered meanings into current existence.

Premises of Hermeneutics

Three premises underlie the application of Hermeneutics. First is the idea of **linguisticality**, or the primacy of language (Gadamer, 1976; Redeker, 1973). Language is not merely words; it also carries tradition, culture, and norms or mores. Hermeneutics is premised upon linguisticality and the idea of *tradition* (see Box 10-1). Finally Hermeneutics invokes the idea of **praxis**, the Greek term for "action," and presented

---

BOX 10-1

PREMISES OF HERMENEUTICS

Linguisticality: the primacy of language
Tradition: culture, norms, history are embedded in language
Praxis: action integrated with knowledge (customary conduct)

in Aristotle's writings as "doing" (in contrast to "making") (Honderich, 1995). In common contemporary use, the term praxis might be defined as "customary conduct." As described in Chapter 9, praxis captures the integration of knowledge and action, rendering the idea of practice as a way of life (Thorne & Hayes, 1996).

Language, in Hermeneutics, is not merely a way of conveying information; it also is a form of expression. Language is a universal phenomenon that can connect people and link past and present. This idea of language can be contrasted with the positivist notion of language as presented in analytic philosophy. Analytic philosophy, in general, was oriented toward breaking things apart to identify constituent components. For the analytic philosophers, words were seen as having a direct relationship to objects. In such an approach, language would be examined (or developed as needed) according to rules of correspondence and prescriptions for the combination of words in a way that would "mirror" reality (Rorty, 1979). Philosophers, in general, use processes of analysis to determine underlying values, definitions, or components of a situation. In contrast, Hermeneutics is an interpretive process aimed at preserving the whole and integrating disparate pieces. The process of philosophical analysis along with the field of epistemology is oriented toward "knowing" and is founded on the idea of a common ground as a basis for judgment: a common language or a common idea of rationality. In contrast, Hermeneutics rejects such a common ground and instead unites people as having differing viewpoints that can enlighten each other (Rorty, 1979).

Being hermeneutical rather than epistemological in thinking requires (or perhaps allows) nurses to recognize that all pursuits do not have to be based on some common ground. Through much of epistemology and especially philosophy of science, the primary concern for a common ground has been the idea of an objective reality and the pursuit of Truth. A hermeneutic philosophy recognizes that popular viewpoints and methods do not have some privileged, unique attachment to reality. Hermeneutics does not separate the world into a realm of facts, where everything that is not a fact is considered a value (Rorty, 1979). Nurses can recognize quite easily that the traditions of knowledge seeking in philosophy and the pursuit of science in other endeavors have been successful to a great extent. The response to that success has been to try to reshape all inquiry to fit this tradition. Doing so, however, does not guarantee continued success or progress; it does provide adherence to existing paradigms and conformity within the prevailing norms. Being hermeneutical in the approach to inquiry acknowledges that current traditions provide only one set of descriptions and one set from a potentially large group of available possible descriptions. In keeping with this idea of alternate descriptions, philosopher Richard Rorty (1979) sees the role for philosophy as changed to "keeping the conversation going" rather than passing judgment on activities. He sees "human beings as generators of new descriptions rather than beings one hopes to be able to describe accurately" (p. 398).

Similar to several other philosophical traditions, Hermeneutics is both a philosophy and a method of inquiry. The two characterizations are inextricably linked; it is not reasonable to attempt to discuss one without the other. Hermeneutics is a way of understanding the world and, as such, entails certain approaches to seeing or reading the world around us. All philosophy carries certain ideas about how to view the world; the line between philosophy and methodology is necessarily a blurry one. It is perhaps a shortcoming of traditional scientific procedures that the philosophy may be more covert with the implications not considered properly or, worse yet, ignored altogether. In the case of Hermeneutics the philosophy and methodology carry the same name and the overlap between the two is particularly apparent.

Hermeneutics is employed to examine the whole expression of a text and the author's meaning. The purpose is to reveal meaning rather than uncover the author's true *intent*. Hermeneutic **interpretation** is a mechanism for "getting behind the surface phenomena and data" (Gadamer, 1981, p. 100). Gadamer (1981) describes the situation encountered in attempts to understand historic texts:

> As soon as one acknowledges that one's own perspective is utterly different from the viewpoints of the authors and the meanings of the texts of the past, there arises the need for a unique effort to avoid misunderstanding the meaning of old texts and yet to comprehend them in their persuasive force. The description of the inner structure and coherence of a given text and the mere repetition of what the author says is not yet real understanding. One has to bring his speaking back to life again, and for this one has to become familiar with the realities about which the text speaks. (p. 98)

This process of bridging the gap between the context of the speaker (producer of the text) and the reader (who is attempting to interpret or understand it) is the central act of hermeneutic understanding.

The Hermeneutic Circle

In determining meaning, the interpreter enters into the interaction with the text with a language that is fraught with tradition. This tradition and other existing prejudices are natural occurrences and constitute a condition of **preunderstanding** according to Gadamer. Some prejudices are "enabling" while others tend to "blind." Preunderstanding is essential in that it enables connection to occur among people in different situations; for example, communication would not be possible without some common language. It also can take on the role of blinding prejudice; however, refining preunderstanding is an important part of the hermeneutic process so that those binding elements are no longer barriers to understanding.

This process moves in a cyclical manner from preunderstanding to understanding to preunderstanding again. As preunderstanding is identified and refined it becomes a new understanding; this revised understanding then serves as the preunderstanding for subsequent situations. In this circular process, the preunderstanding or prejudices are revised continually until there is the **"fusion of horizons"** between the interpreter and the originator of the text (Gadamer, 1976).

This circular process from preunderstanding to understanding is Gadamer's version of the "**Hermeneutic Circle**" and provides a description of the practice of understanding. The more common form of the hermeneutic circle addresses the way in which interpretation is conducted from the standpoint of how to examine a **text**. Schleiermacher (Redeker, 1973) described a process of proceeding from parts of a text to the whole then reexamining the parts in light of the whole. This process continues until understanding is achieved. The parts include the grammatical components, or the specific language and how it is used in the text. The whole, when viewed in hermeneutic interpretation, takes on a technical or psychological focus, dealing with the author's individual style in using language to express experience and thought. The grammatical component includes each word, sentence, and section as it belongs to the whole. The technical or psychological focus requires the interpreter to penetrate the message of the work by looking at the author's distinctive use of language including organization of the text and, if possible, motive. These two components are highly interrelated; one aspect can be examined only in regard to the other. The interpreter thus follows the hermeneutic circle by working from whole to parts to whole again to uncover meaning in the text.

Ricoeur and the Role of Action

French philosopher Paul Ricoeur added an interesting twist to the development of hermeneutics. Ricoeur (1981) assumes the "primary sense of the word 'hermeneutics' concerns the rules required for the interpretation of the written documents of our culture" (p. 197). He argues that the same principles of hermeneutic interpretation could be applied to action as well as to discourse or written text. Ricoeur discusses **action** as capable of being objectified in a manner similar to the fixation of speech through writing. **Speech** is "exteriorized" through the act of writing, transforming the speech to an external form where it becomes an object amenable to study. According to Ricoeur, action "has the structure of a locutionary act" including propositional content (p. 204). Similar to the act of speech, actions are detached from the performer "in the same way that a text is detached from its author" (p. 206). Action also has relevance and importance that may extend past the immediate situation. Finally action has an audience that may be extensive, just as text has an array of possible readers.

Ricoeur follows the tradition of some poststructuralists in seeing a text as a "work" (Ricoeur, 1981, pp. 136–138). Viewing something as a "work," rather than, in the case of writing, a mere written text, compels the interpreter or reader to view the item (the "work") in its entirety, as a "structured totality which cannot be reduced to the sentences whereof it is composed" (Thompson, 1985, p. 13). Ricoeur (1981) also emphasizes the idea of "distanciation" to capture the idea of the text as removed or distant from normal discourse. The "work" is separate from the original "meaning" or intent of the speaker/writer and stands available to audiences that were not initially intended or known (pp. 142–144). Structural analysis alone cannot render an understanding because it does not reveal the world disclosed by the text. By applying this same idea of distanciation to action, Ricoeur extends the reach of interpretation to the social sciences, arguing that action serves as a suitable text for analysis as well as written language (Ricoeur, 1981; Thompson, 1981).

Hermeneutics and Phenomenology

There has been considerable discussion in the literature of the relationship between hermeneutics and phenomenology particularly in regard to the "idealism" of Husserl and Heidegger. Heidegger relied on many principles of the early work in hermeneutics and adopted much of its terminology. Central to Heidegger's philosophy, for example, are the ideas of understanding and interpretation. Heidegger, however, focused on the individual Being and argued for techniques to disclose the "basic existential structures of human existence" (Mueller-Vollmer, 1988, p. 34), which Heidegger referred to as *Dasein* (Heidegger, 1962). Heidegger advanced the idea of the hermeneutic circle and the roles of preunderstanding and understanding, which were expanded later by Gadamer, and similarly emphasized the linguistic nature of human experience (Heidegger, 1962, 1971).

Heidegger may be most closely associated with the tradition of existentialism in philosophy and with phenomenology. His influence on hermeneutics, however, provided a blending of both existentialism and phenomenology. "Heideggerian Hermeneutics" seems to be the form of hermeneutic interpretation most commonly used in nursing inquiry. Benner (1984) is credited with introducing this methodology to nursing through her seminal work on practice and expertise (Diekelmann, 1992). Diekelmann has applied Heideggerian hermeneutics using a multi-step process of analysis to understand the "lived experience" of teachers and students in various learning situations. Such work helps to reveal the "narratives" that exist in the lives of people and creates new ways of viewing situations. In the study of Learning-as-Testing, for example, Diekelmann (1992) provides new insights into the traditional approach to education, revealing the primary themes that reflect how such situations are constituted and lived. Typically in such research, participants are encouraged simply to relate what happened along with their thoughts and feelings rather than provide an analytic or explanatory account of their experiences. Striving for new understanding of the situation in its totality, the research aims to interpret the resulting text. This aim differentiates hermeneutics and other methods that may be referred to as interpretive from other forms of qualitative research. Other researchers have employed hermeneutic methods to explore various aspects of nursing practice (Cronin, 2001; Cutcliffe, 1999, Milligan, 2001; Nelms, 1996; Nystrom, Dahlberg, & Carlsson, 2003; Walters, 1996), learning situations (Jordan, 1996; Little, 1999), and illness experiences (Dzurec, 1994; Sundin, Jansson, & Norberg, 2002). Hermeneutic approaches to inquiry also are found in the Steeves' (1992) work with bone marrow transplantation recipients and in his studies with other researchers into the experiences of suffering (Steeves, Kahn, & Benoliel, 1990).

CRITICAL SOCIAL THEORY

Critical theory, or **Critical Social Theory**, as it most commonly is implemented, offers another philosophical tradition of interest and relevance to nursing knowledge. Critical Social Theory is characterized by an emphasis on language, power relations, and the social processes associated with knowledge. Critical theory in general advocates that doctrines and knowledge claims are products of social processes and must be examined to identify implicit origins and ideologies. The emerging dominance of technology at the time of its development as a view of knowledge was a particularly strong impetus for examining the roles and outcomes of science (see Box 10-2).

Critical Social Theory, like Hermeneutics, falls within the postmodern tradition and shares the European background of other leading philosophies of the time. Critical theory originated in what is referred to as the **Frankfurt School**. This group was associated with the formation of the Institute for Social Research, a group of radical thinkers in Frankfurt, Germany. Max Horkheimer assumed the position of director of the Institute in 1931, and the basic premises of critical theory soon began to emerge. The work was stimulated by Marxist theory, the social and political developments of the time, and scholars such as Horkheimer, Adorno, and Marcuse (Horkheimer & Adorno, 1972).

The Contributions of Habermas

In contemporary contexts, the most commonly used approach to critical theory was developed by Jürgen Habermas, who represents a later wave of rejuvenation of work in this area. Habermas varied from the original ideas of critical theory in the Frankfurt School by decreasing the emphasis on Marxist philosophy and ideas of political oppression and increasing the focus on human social interaction on a broad level. His Theory of **Communicative Action** presents a view that goes beyond the critique of ideology proposed by the Frankfurt School. Instead he advocates for communication that involves all interested persons in exchange free of any dominating influence.

BOX 10-2

PREMISES OF CRITICAL SOCIAL THEORY

Knowledge claims reflect social processes.
Language takes a primary role.
Power is reflected in knowledge claims.
Understanding requires awareness of the origins and ideologies reflected in
    knowledge claims.

Habermas (1971) tied his ideas closely to social science and to philosophy. The "theory of knowledge" or "epistemology" has a long tradition in philosophy in spite of the diversion created by the advent of modern science. Habermas (1971) argued that, somewhere along the line, "philosophy's position regard to science . . . [had] been undermined by the movement of philosophical thought itself" (p. 4). The theory of knowledge was "replaced by a methodology emptied of philosophical thought" (p. 4). "Scientism" emerged, with science believing in "its exclusive validity..." (p. 4). Recognizing the indisputable success of Positivism, Habermas embarked on an exploration of the context of its development, moving to a critique of epistemology particularly from the standpoint of human interests.

Habermas' (1971) view of knowledge is most easily understood by examining his distinctions among three categories of inquiry: the empirical-analytic, the historical-hermeneutic, and the critical (p. 308). According to Habermas (1971), the empirical-analytic sciences provide rules for construction and testing of theory. The hypothetico-deductive approach (see Chapter 6) enables the development of laws and propositions that ultimately enable prediction of events. Habermas describes this approach as bearing a "cognitive interest in technical control over objectified processes" (p. 309).

The historical-hermeneutic sciences reflect an interest that is *practical* in contrast to the *technical* interest of the empirical-analytic model. In these sciences, the interpretation of texts is at the center of the process and rules deal with understanding and meaning rather than observation of empirical phenomena. Habermas takes exception with the premise of the hermeneutic philosophers who make it appear "as though the interpreter transposes himself into the horizon of the world or language from which a text derives its meaning" (p. 309). This is an illusion, Habermas contends, as this approach has a self-validating frame of reference. As Habermas argues, "the facts first are constituted in relation to the standards that establish them" (p. 309).

Finally Habermas identifies the category of the *sciences of social action*. These sciences, economics, political science, and sociology, have the same general goal as the empirical-analytic sciences. The *critical* social science goes further, however, to determine the possible roles of ideology in that knowledge. The primary methodology is grounded in self-reflection and based on a primary cognitive interest in *emancipation* (p. 310). Habermas concludes that human beings attempt to grasp reality from three distinct viewpoints and their related "categories of possible knowledge":

> information that expands our power of technical control; interpretations that make possible the orientation of action within common traditions; and analyses that free consciousness from its dependence of hypostatized powers. These viewpoints originate in the interest structure of a species that is linked in its roots to definite means of social organization: work, language, and power. (p. 313)

Habermas places his philosophical position within the domain of the other "sciences" yet moves beyond the other forms of knowledge and understanding to emancipation from the structures, ideologies, and power systems that exist.

Habermas' Theory of Communicative Action

Consistent with a postmodern emphasis on language and discourse, Habermas also has a strong reliance on aspects of communication throughout his work. This is particularly evident in his theory of "communicative action" (Habermas, 1984). Habermas sees **speech** as existing in various forms, each of which has a different relationship to truth and knowledge. **Communicative action** is not aimed at the imparting of truth or knowledge or the regulation of behavior; it is premised upon the development of mutual understanding among participants in the interaction. The "ideal speech situation" provides the opportunity for all participants equally to express their desires and viewpoints and both to challenge and articulate the validity of truth claims in the speech act (Habermas, 1984). According to Habermas, free and equal exchange of ideas is essential to the development of understanding.

Habermas' Critical Social Theory has considerable similarity with Foucault's poststructuralist approach in regard to the existence of power relationships. Foucault, however, focused on the relationship between discourse and knowledge/power and the ways in which certain forms of discourse present a hegemonic perspective, in other words, the perspective of the dominant group. Drawing some of his views from Marx and ideology of oppression, Habermas looks more at experience and interaction but moves beyond this basis to a broader look at society and human interaction. The goal of "emancipation" in Critical Social Theory reveals the action-oriented approach of this view (Habermas, 1984), emancipating groups from oppressive ideologies rather than merely improving understanding through recognition of the power relationships that exist.

Both Hermeneutics and Critical Social Theory share the postmodern antifoundationist perspective. In other words, these traditions do not subscribe to the idea that there is an objective "foundation" that can be used as a point of reference or a criterion to evaluate knowledge claims. Knowledge instead has a strong human element in that it is primarily a social construction.[1] As Allen, Benner and Diekelmann (1986) describe this situation,

> the criteria that scientists (or anyone) use to separate knowledge from fiction or mere belief are always based on social conventions, on a negotiated agreement, not on some transcendental appeal to "facts" against which one can supposedly measure the validity of an assertion. (p. 33)

---

[1]This position often is referred to as Constructivism, the idea that people "construct" their own individual realities.

Rationality continues to be a strong focus in Critical Social Theory but not the rationality of "science." Instead rationality exists where there is free and equal expression and positions and viewpoints can be expressed without coercion or fear of reprisal (Habermas, 1984).

IMPLICATIONS FOR NURSING

The postmodern approaches to inquiry reflect a variety of goals ranging from knowledge to enlightenment and ultimately "emancipation." These approaches to inquiry represent a shift from "science" exemplified by theory or paradigm development to edification and alternative ways of viewing the world. These approaches reflect what has been termed a "human science" approach in contrast to the natural sciences supported by empiricism.

All these views emphasize the human element in knowledge. Language takes a central role: as a tool for conveying tradition, norms, and mores, in addition to reflecting social hierarchies and relationships. As a discipline, nursing has long espoused a strong emphasis on personal interaction. A nurse aspires to "know" the patient (client) and work *with* the patient in a collaborative manner to arrive at mutually acceptable goals and actions.

The concept of "person" always has occupied the center of nursing's knowledge base. One challenge in knowledge development has been to focus on the person as the center of nursing attention without objectifying the individual. In other words, nurses need knowledge about human beings for developing the knowledge base as well as for providing care for the individual. Yet it is not consistent with the espoused ethics of nursing to view the human as an object to be acted upon.

Hermeneutics and Critical Social Theory place the person at the front of the inquiry or interaction. In patient care, hermeneutics recognizes that people have different experiences and perspectives. As a result, the nurse cannot assume that he or she necessarily understands the person's viewpoint in spite of whatever commonalities the nurse and the patient may share. A hermeneutic approach compels the nurse to recognize that each individual has a unique reality constructed by culture, language, and tradition. Individual biases and "preunderstanding" can be both blinding and enabling in the attempt to understand the experiences and viewpoint of others.

Hermeneutic inquiry seems wholly consistent with nursing's attempt to maintain recognition of the person. The idea of people as "embodied" has become more commonplace in recent discussions. This notion of the "embodied self" stands in direct contrast to Cartesian dualism that supported mental and physical realms as distinct. People's lives have been regarded as narratives (MacIntyre, 1984; Ricoeur, 1984) with each life constructed as a different story. This view opens personal identity and experience as a story or narrative that can be interpreted.

Hermeneutic methods provide the opportunity for a deeper appreciation of human experience. Rather than reducing aspects of individual behavior to a level of law-like causality, a hermeneutic approach enables a stronger awareness of individuals' perceptions. Such awareness gives the nurse the sensitivity that is vital to form an effective health promoting relationships. Many situations encountered by nurse do not require "intervention" or some action to "fix" the current situation. Instead the nurse may be most in need of the awareness and understanding provided through interpretive inquiry. Without a doubt, such understanding is the cornerstone of any effective intervention or interaction.

Nurses are not excluded from having a major role in the power dynamics of health care situations in regard to their own status in institutions and their position of apparent power over individual recipients of care. In many nursing encounters, effective work with a patient or client requires reflection and self-awareness. Dealing with complex systems such as health care and vast bodies of commonly espoused "knowledge" puts both patients and nurses at risk for being swept up in dominant ideology. Persons outside the dominant mainstream may not be aware of a full range of treatment options or may not feel empowered to contribute to their own care and planning. The areas of transcultural care and women's health have provided considerable information revealing the potential for oppression and less than optimal care as a result of existing power structures in health care (Dickson, 1990). Effective and appropriate care may be premised on a need, first, to recognize the existence of such power dynamics. Then the individual can be assisted to realize the nature of the interaction and be empowered to take a more active role in care or to seek alternatives.

Critical Social Theory also can be applicable to gaining a new perspective on the nurses' own situation. Changes in practice and in environmental design could take place without involvement of the people affected by the changes, for example, nurses and patients. Computer documentation programs may be developed without review and participation by nurses (Moen, Henry, & Warren, 1999) resulting in cumbersome systems that decrease efficiency and morale. The design of a nursing unit and work areas without any lounge, break, or other private space fails to recognize nurses' needs for occasional time where they are not on view or could use a quiet work space. Inquiry that sheds light on the nature of relationships in times of institutional change can empower all parties to be more active participants.

Action research bears some similarity to the processes of Critical Social Theory. In action research (Argyris, Putnam, & Smith, 1985; Carr & Kemmis, 1986; Whyte, 1991), the investigator is an active group member who brings about change along with the other participants. Consider, for example, a situation where several residents in a community want to decrease the use of lawn herbicides and pesticides. A nurse could provide educational materials or programs or leaflets for distribution. In such a situation the nurse stands in a position of distant authority, informing the public but not really involved or invested in their activities or outcomes. As an alternative, the nurse might choose to become an active participant in the group, providing information and expertise yet contributing along with the other members to achieve mutually desired results. In an action research model, the nurse also could be in the role of investigator, exploring processes of leadership and change while promoting and evaluating movement toward outcomes.

Holter & Kim (1995) compare the traditional notion of action research derived from a natural science perspective with a critical action perspective. A striking difference between the two is the collaboration between the researcher and those being studied and the importance of mutual understanding in the critical approach. In critical action research, the researcher and the other participants mutually determine activity goals; the researcher does not impose the goals. The researcher's idea of a healthy community cannot be conveyed to participants, but must be arrived at through engagement and understanding. In a natural science perspective, procedures may be more one sided with the researcher having a more authoritative role in setting goals for the encounter.

 ## CONCLUSION

The interpretive methods offer nurses new ways of seeing familiar situations and new ideas for inquiry. Knowledge is entrenched clearly as a human development: knowledge always is the knowledge *of* someone; it is not an autonomous object to be found and documented. Methods derived from such approaches require reconsideration of ways of determining quality and credibility because the traditional foundationist perspective is not applicable. Continuing development of philosophy in this area and associated methodologies is likely to give nurses many alternatives for inquiry in the future.

 ## FOR DISCUSSION

1. Discuss the basic tenets of the philosophies of Hermeneutics and Critical Social Theory.
2. Discuss the nature of "truth" as it pertains to the philosophical traditions of Hermeneutics and Critical Social Theory.
3. Compare and contrast the philosophies of Hermeneutics and Critical Social Theory in regard to traditional ideas about "science." How would work using a methodology based on one of these philosophies compare to common ideas about science?

4. Identify criteria that might be useful to evaluate the quality of inquiry based on the philosophy of Hermeneutics or Critical Social Theory.

5. Discuss strengths and limitations of these philosophical traditions in regard to the development of nursing knowledge.

REFERENCES

Allen, D., Benner, P., & Diekelmann, N. (1986). Three paradigms for nursing research: Methodological implications. In P. L. Chinn, *Nursing research methodology: Issues and implementation* (pp. 23–38). Rockville, MD: Aspen.

Argyris, C., Putnam, R., & Smith, D. M. (1985). *Action science: Concepts, methods and skills for research and intervention*. San Francisco, CA.: Jossey-Bass.

Benner, P. (1984). From novice to expert : Excellence and power in clinical nursing practice. Menlo Park, CA: Addison-Wesley.Publishing.

Carr, W., & Kemmis, S. (1986). *Becoming critical: Education knowledge and action research*. London: Falmer Press.

Cassirer, E. (1944). *An essay on man: An introduction to a philosophy of human culture*. New Haven, CT: Yale University Press.

Cronin, C. (2001). How do nurses deal with their emotions on a burn unit? A hermeneutic inquiry. *Journal of Clinical Nursing, 10*, 301–302.

Cutcliffe, J. R. (1999). Qualified nurses' lived experience of violence perpetrated by individuals suffering from enduring mental health problems: A hermeneutic study. *International Journal of Nursing Studies, 36*, 105–116.

Derrida, J. (1974). *Of grammatology* (G. C. Spivak, Trans.). Baltimore: Johns Hopkins University Press.

Dickson, G. L. (1990). A feminist poststructuralist analysis of the knowledge of menopause. *Advances in Nursing Science, 12*(3), 15–31.

Diekelmann, N. L. (1992). Learning-as-testing: A Heideggerian hermeneutical analysis of the lived experiences of students and teachers in nursing. *Advances in Nursing Science, 14*(3), 72–83.

Dilthey, W. (1976). *Selected writings* (H. P. Rickman, Ed. & Trans.). Cambridge: Cambridge University Press.

Droysen, J. G. (1977). *Outline of the principles of history* (E. B. Andrews, Trans.). Boston: Ginn & Co.

Dzurec, L. C. (1994). Schizophrenic clients' experiences of power: Using hermeneutic analysis. *Image: Journal of Nursing Scholarship, 26*, 155–159.

Gadamer, H. (1975). *Truth and method* (G. Barden & J. Cumming, Trans.). New York: Seabury Press.

Gadamer, H. (1976). On the scope and function of hermeneutical reflection (G. B. Hess & R. E. Palmer, Trans.). In D. E. Linge (Ed.), *Philosophical hermeneutics* (pp. 18–43). Berkeley: University of California Press.

Gadamer, H. (1981). *Reason in the age of science*. (F. G. Lawrence, Trans.). Cambridge, MA: MIT Press.

Habermas, J. (1971). *Knowledge and human interests*. Boston: Beacon Press.

Habermas, J. (1984). *Theory of communicative action* (2 vols). (T. McCarthy, Trans.). Boston: Beacon Press.

Heidegger, M. (1962). *Being and time*. (J. Macquarrie & E. Robinson, Trans.). New York: Harper.

Heidegger, M. (1971). *On the way to language*. (P. D. Hertz, Trans.). New York: Harper & Row.

Holter, I. M., & Kim, H. S. (1995). Methodology for critical theory: Critical action research. In A. Omery, C. E. Kasper, & G. G. Page (Eds.), *In search of nursing science* (pp. 220–232). Thousand Oaks, CA: Sage Publications.

Honderich, T. (Ed.). (1995). *The Oxford companion to philosophy*. Oxford: Oxford University Press.

Horkheimer, M., & Adorno, T. (1972). *Dialectic of enlightenment* (J. Cumming, Trans.). New York: Seabury.

Humboldt, W. von (1963). *Humanist without portfolio: An anthology of the writings of Wilhelm von Humboldt* (M. Cowan, Trans.). Detroit, MI: Wayne State University Press.

Husserl, E. (1970). *The crisis of European sciences and transcendental phenomenology: An introduction to phenomenological philosophy* (D. Carr, Trans.). Evanston, IL: Northwestern University Press.

Jordan, J. D. (1996). Rethinking race and attrition in nursing programs: A hermeneutic inquiry. *Journal of Professional Nursing, 12,* 382–390.

Kant, I. (1965). *Critique of pure reason* (N. K. Smith, Trans.). New York: St. Martin's Press.

Little, C. V. (1999). The meaning of learning in critical care nursing: A hermeneutic study. *Journal of Advanced Nursing, 30,* 697–703.

MacIntyre, A. (1984). *After virtue: A study in moral theory* (2nd Ed). Notre Dame, IN: University of Notre Dame Press.

Milligan, F. (2001). The concept of care in male nurse work: An ontological hermeneutic study in acute hospitals. *Journal of Advanced Nursing, 35,* 7–16.

Moen, A., Henry, S. B., & Warren, J. J. (1999). Representing nursing judgements in the electronic health record. *Journal of Advanced Nursing, 30,* 990–997.

Mueller-Vollmer, K. (Ed.). (1988). *The hermeneutics reader.* New York: Continuum.

Nelms, T. P. (1996). Living a caring presence in nursing: A Heideggerian hermeneutical analysis. *Journal of Advanced Nursing, 24,* 368–374.

Nystrom, M., Dahlberg, K., & Carlsson, G. (2003). Non-caring encounters at an emergency care unit— a life-world hermeneutic analysis of an efficiency-driven organization. *International Journal of Nursing Studies, 40,* 761–769.

Redeker, M. (1973). *Schleiermacher: Life and thought.* (J. Walihausser, Trans). Philadelphia: Fortress Press.

Ricoeur, P. (1981). *Hermeneutics and the human sciences* (J. B. Thompson, Ed. and Trans.). Cambridge: Cambridge University Press.

Ricoeur, P. (1984). *Time and narrative* (2 vols). (K. McLaughlin & D. Pellauer, Trans.). Chicago: University of Chicago Press.

Rorty, R. (1979). *Philosophy and the mirror of nature.* Princeton: Princeton University Press.

Steeves, R. H. (1992). Patients who have undergone bone marrow transplantation: their quest for meaning. *Oncology Nursing Forum, 19,* 899–905.

Steeves, R. H., Kahn, D. L., & Benoliel, J. Q. (1990). Nurses' interpretation of the suffering of their patients. *Western Journal of Nursing Research, 12,* 715–729.

Sundin, K., Jansson, L., & Norberg, A. (2002). Understanding between care providers and patients with stroke and aphasia: A phenomenological hermeneutic inquiry. *Nursing Inquiry, 9,* 93–103.

Thompson, J. L. (1985). Practical discourse in nursing: Going beyond empiricism and historicism. *Advances in Nursing Science, 7*(4), 59–71.

Thorne, S. E., & Hayes, V. E. (Ed.). (1996). *Nursing praxis: Knowledge and action.* Thousand Oaks, CA: Sage Publications.

Walters, A. J. (1996). Being a clinical nurse consultant: A hermeneutic phenomenological reflection. *International Journal of Nursing Practice, 2*(1), 2–10.

Whyte, W. F. (1991). *Participatory action research.* Newbury Park, CA: Sage.

Feminism and Science

Feminism is a relatively new addition to the literature of philosophy and research methods, gaining increasing attention through the latter part of the 20th century. The development of feminist epistemology was made possible by the rise of postmodernism. This philosophy recognized that social structures and classes could have a significant influence on knowledge claims. Postmodernists had worked to erase the previous divide between the "knower" and the "known," showing how the person or group of people responsible for creating the knowledge had some effect on its construction. Gender can be an important element in shaping knowledge as well as in the constructing individual experiences.

THE BEGINNINGS OF FEMINIST POLITICS

Combined with a growing feminist interest, the philosophy of postmodernism made it evident that women essentially had been excluded from much research.

For the most part, women were not involved in doing the research and also tended to be excluded from studies as subjects. Issues related to access to women as subjects, childbearing ability and accompanying risks, and hormonal fluctuation could complicate attempts to conduct "controlled" studies and increase the costs associated with conducting research.[1] Women also tended not to pursue careers in the sciences, so their opinions were minimal or not heard in designing and conducting research. Recognition of these situations in the development of knowledge provided a context for the consideration of inquiry that was not only *about* women but conducted *for* women (often by women) and, by extension, from the perspective of women.

The distinction among types of research as being *about* or *for* women or conducted *from the perspective of* women parallels two major elements of **feminism** in regard to knowledge development. One aspect of feminism considers gender as a variable, for example, the experiences of women compared to those of men, women's moral development or caregiving needs compared to men's, and cardiac symptoms of women differing from those of men. Such research provides valuable information about women in a variety of social settings and medical conditions. Not surprisingly, much of this type of research completed to date has brought attention to the significant limitations associated with results of studies based on males when those results are extrapolated to the population of women.

Beyond the obvious physiologic uniqueness of women, feminism has become of interest in nursing particularly for its emphasis on sociological aspects associated with being female. Feminist scholars vary in the intensity of their arguments, yet there is general agreement that women occupy a unique position in societies. Oppression has been associated with the lack of legislated rights as well as to a general patriarchal social structure that grants higher status to the males in a culture. Feminist scholars may espouse ideology ranging anywhere from a general liberal sense to a Marxist or radical Marxist ideology depending on the degree of discrimination envisioned and the sources of oppression and discrimination.

Other scholars see the world primarily as androcentric, meaning it is based on males as the center and a male worldview. In such a view, social structures and economic classes favor males, putting them automatically in positions of authority and dominance by mere virtue of their being male. For such scholars, a feminist approach means adopting a different balance and focus and, as a result, different forms of inquiry.

---

[1]The National Institutes of Health implemented guidelines in 1994 specifically mandating the inclusion of women and minorities in NIH-funded research. These guidelines were consistent with the NIH Revitalization Act of 1993, Public Law (PL) 103-43. The guidelines have been updated numerous times since the original position was published in the NIH Guide for Grants and Contracts, Vol. 19, No. 31, August 24, 1990 and Vol. 19, No. 35, September 28, 1990. The most recent guidelines dated October 9, 2001 are available at the NIH web site, http://grants2.nih.gov/grants/guide/notice-files/NOT-OD-02-001.html (accessed March 20, 2004).

The important point to be recognized from this initial introduction is that feminism has a long and varied history although its emergence in the literature of epistemology is more recent. Feminism means very different things to different people, and the simple labeling of an approach as "feminist" may not reveal a great deal about the inquiry or its philosophical underpinnings. Feminism's nature as both philosophical and political further complicates its understanding; varying degrees of each aspect are apparent in any particular situation.

It is, therefore, potentially misleading to discuss such a thing as feminism as if it were one distinguishable body. It is not a solitary or unified philosophy nor is there a single feminist viewpoint. In this chapter, examination of feminism is oriented toward providing some understanding of features that are generally shared under the heading of feminism while simultaneously building awareness of the wide range of ideology that may fall under this subject.

Seneca Falls Convention of 1848

All feminism shares a grounding in politics devoted to advancing the status of women. While feminism may mean a number of different things philosophically, it is inherently political. Therefore, a reasonable starting point for discussion of feminism is with a brief overview of feminism as a political movement.

Feminism as a political movement has a lengthy history in social development dating at least to the 14th century and proceeding to the present. In contemporary Western societies, the Seneca Falls Convention of 1848 is considered the landmark event in the development of the political movement. Elizabeth Cady Stanton, a major figure in the women's political movement, met Lucretia Mott in London in 1840 when they both attended the World Anti-Slavery Convention. Ironically the conference had refused seating to Stanton and Mott along with other female attendees because they were women. The idea developed that a convention should be held to address the plight of women. The Seneca Falls Convention occurred eight years later as a rather serendipitous event. Stanton wrote a Declaration of Sentiments to serve as a focal point for the convention. The Declaration of Independence was used to provide a basic format for the declaration, and Stanton's work was premised on the principle that all men *and women* had been created equal. The role of men, particularly in their actions toward women, was given the same review as the King of England toward the colonists including a "long train of abuses and usurpations" (Stanton, 1889). Stanton concluded the Declaration as follows:

> Now, in view of this entire disenfranchisement of one-half the people of this country, their social and religious degradation—in view of the unjust laws above mentioned and because women do feel themselves aggrieved, oppressed, and fraudulently deprived of their most sacred rights, we insist that they have immediate admission to all the rights and privileges which belong to them as citizens of the United States. (p. 70)

One hundred women and men signed the Declaration. Ten resolutions associated with this document were passed by unanimous vote at the convention. An eleventh resolution supporting that women should work to secure the right of women to vote also passed but after considerable debate and without a unanimous vote. By 1920 when women actually did receive the right to vote, only one of the original signers of the Declaration at Seneca Falls had survived to cast her vote (Smithsonian Institution, 2003). Recognition of issues associated with gender has persisted since this monumental beginning. More recently, political effort has focused on equal access and opportunities for women in all arenas including pay equity, academics and sports, job security, and flexibility to meet the challenges of various family situations such as child rearing and elder caregiving. A constitutional amendment guaranteeing equal rights for women has been debated since the 1970s but has not been ratified by the necessary number of states to enact this constitutional change.

FEMINIST PHILOSOPHY

Regardless of the degree of passion for social reform or the meaning attached to gender in philosophy and science, feminist viewpoints seem to have at least one element in common. That element concerns the idea of a dominant patriarchy and the importance of political action to counteract the dominant hegemony. Feminist philosophy presents a woman-centered view as an alternative to androcentric or male-centered philosophical, social, and cultural tradition. As noted previously, much biological and medical research had been standardized as a result of studies with subjects who were male. Often results were misapplied because they were not applicable to women's unique physiology and experiences (see Box 11-1).

Equally as often, women were judged to be inferior as a way of explaining identified differences in results obtained from separate studies of women and men. One of the most frequently cited examples of the presumed inferiority of women comes from the work of Kohlberg on human and moral development. In his classic work on moral development, Kohlberg (1981; Power, Higgins-D'Alessan-

---

BOX 11-1

BASIC TENETS OF FEMINIST PHILOSOPHY

- Science is inherently gendered.
- Society and science reflect the dominant patriarchy and androcentric bias.
- Woman-centered view is an appropriate alternative to androcentric philosophy and social and cultural traditions.
- Feminism is dedicated to advancing the status of women.

dro, & Kohlberg, 1989) identified various stages of development and presented strategies for assisting students to achieve higher levels of the development. Application of aspects of Kohlberg's model revealed that female students were at a considerably different (i.e., lower) level of development when compared to males. According to this study, females appeared to be intellectually and morally less developed or less mature. Gilligan (1982) raised questions about Kohlberg's studies, pointing out that tests reflected the performance of males and might not be valid when applied to females. When she studied moral problem solving in girls and women, she found a substantially different orientation to problems in her sample. The ethical problems were framed differently by the females; in other words, the key components and central issues were viewed differently. As a result, problem-solving techniques differed. This was a reflection of a different frame of reference, not a higher or lower level of moral development.

Building on this work, Belenky et al. (1986) conducted in-depth interviews with 135 women, 90 of whom were recent alumnae or current students and another 45 women recruited through family agencies. The results of their study revealed that women had ways of interacting with and knowing the world that were substantively different from those of men. A patriarchal view of knowledge allows for only one way of gaining knowledge, that which is consistent with the intellectual processes of men. Other ways of viewing the world are either suppressed or denigrated.

Feminism argues that science is inherently gendered not only for its treatment of women or failure to incorporate women as subjects for study but also for its exclusive views of what counts as science. A critical point in feminist philosophy in regard to science concerns this presumed androcentric bias. This bias is purported to be evident not only in how results of science are applied but in the ontological perspective offered. In other words, an androcentric bias would be reflected in the general assumptions about how reality exists. Keller (1983a) describes the status of science and particularly the idea of objectivity as essentially masculine. The separation of the knower from the known, which reflects the objectivity imperative in traditional science, calls upon specific methodologies or interactions to unite these two aspects of existence. Reason and logic serve as the medium of knowledge not emotion or feeling. Science also is considered to reflect a masculine bias in references to nature as female and something to be controlled or conquered.[1]

Philosopher Sandra Harding (1986) differentiated three forms of feminism: Feminist empiricism, Feminist standpoint, and Feminist postmodernism. **Feminist empiricism** advocates a more equitable and inclusive approach to traditional science. According to this view, a restricted perspective is the primary problem confronted by science. A feminist approach provides a broader perspective and thus actually enhances rather than threatens existing science (Harding, 1986, p. 24–25). Feminist researchers engaging in feminist empiricism may not see themselves as

---

[1]The Freudian implications of references to gender identity here are noteworthy. Keller (1983b) captures some of this emphasis, as well as that of other developmental psychologists in her discussion of the formation of identity.

BOX 11-2

FORMS OF FEMINISM (HARDING, 1991)

+ **Feminist Empiricism.** This view preserves existing methodology and rules of science.

+ **Feminist Standpoint.** The view of women in the construction of knowledge has advantages over the view of men.

+ **Feminist Postmodernism.** There is no singular human experience (no metanarrative); human experience varies according to a variety of factors including social status, ethnicity, and gender among others.

---

doing feminist research. Instead "they see themselves as primarily following more rigorously the existing rules and principles of the sciences" (Harding, 1991, p. 111). Box 11-2 outlines several forms of feminist philosophy.

Feminist empiricism preserves the "existing methodological norms" (Harding, 1986, p. 25) and as a result presents a view that is more likely to be acceptable in mainstream science. However, Harding (1991) finds numerous problems with feminist empiricism that limit its effectiveness. A primary problem concerns the situation resulting from feminist empiricism's major strength. Feminist empiricism claims that the traditional implementation of the scientific method is responsible for introducing bias in science yet it supports those methods as appropriate for rigorous science. According to Harding, those very rules and norms of science are responsible for the existing androcentric bias. The inclusion of women scientists with a feminist viewpoint will not alter the conduct of science as long as the traditional methods are preserved.

The **feminist standpoint** holds that the viewpoint of women is a "morally and scientifically preferable grounding for our interpretations and explanations of nature and social life" (Harding, 1986, p. 26). Feminist standpoint holds that the researcher's gender and social status influence the conduct and results of inquiry. This position is premised on the idea that men hold a dominant position in the human social order and that this vantage point results in "partial and perverse understandings" (p. 26). Women's position, in contrast, "provides the possibility of more complete and less perverse understandings" (p. 26).

Harding acknowledges the temptation of **relativism**, that is, the idea that knowledge claims must be considered in relation (or relative to) particular contexts, in considering the preceding two forms of feminist thought. Relativism, however, places various positions on equal footing, as being equally defensible and worthy. While there is room for debate as well as refinement of these views, this is not consistent with philosophical relativism. As Allen (1992) points out, feminists believe that the feminist view is a preferable option not "just an alternative

Knowledg is contextual

to racism, sexism, or classism" (p. 1). The need for further refinement actually is a condition of all science (Harding, 1986, p. 27) and imperfections in feminist views need to be viewed as appropriate within the context of any science.

One criticism of the preceding views concerns the apparent position that there is a single women's view. The experiences of women may vary in response to the influence of factors such as race and class. In essence, it is questionable whether any one view or "set of rules" can reflect the experiences of women (Harding, 1986, pp. 26–27). This point leads to a criticism levied by **feminist postmodernism**, the final form of feminism described by Harding. This form acknowledges the "fractured identities" that exist in contemporary societies where social status, political identity, and ethnicity as only a few examples counteract the idea of a singular human experience. Harding adds that this singular "human" experience commonly reflects what she calls the "manly" experience (p. 28).

Recognition that women hold a marginalized position in many ways in regard to science mirrors the absence or silence of other oppressed groups. In response, new areas of study have emerged that "give voice" to the members of such groups. Women's studies was one of the first of these areas to emerge and seek legitimacy in academic settings. A scholarly focus also has emerged to address the unique perspectives of various other ethnic and cultural or social groups. Study in such fields aims to counteract the presumed white male centered view that ordinarily pervades history as well as current thought. Although concerned particularly with the situation of women, feminist postmodernism invites alternative perspectives that address the world views of other similarly excluded groups.

OUTCOMES OF FEMINIST PHILOSOPHY

Feminist philosophy obviously can take various forms. One outcome can be the education and training of more women as "scientists." A presumption seems to be that the mere presence of women in science brings another perspective to scientific endeavors that will enhance the work. Such positions give credence to the idea that there are natural inherent gender differences and that these differences result in varying frames of reference associated with the diversity among scientists.

One general difference that accompanies gender is associated with the ways in which males and females relate to the world and to other beings. Carol Gilligan's (1982) respondents acted more from an understanding of complex relationships in identifying moral dilemmas and in their approaches to problem solving. This perspective was contrasted with the viewpoint of males, which was driven by a perceived hierarchy of values and principles. Harding (1991) and Keller (1983b) both cite the work of Barbara McClintock and Rachel Carson in their discussions of feminist science, both of which presumably give examples of a more relational approach to the world. McClintock achieved prominence for her work with the genetics of corn, particularly her recognition of how genes can change position along a chromosome.[1] Carson (1941, 1962) is well known for her development of a general ecology and her arguments against pesticide use and environmental pollution. All these examples reveal what these feminist philosophers refer to as a "feminine" ontology as reflected in a "feminist" science.

As these examples illustrate, the "feminist" view sees the elements of the world as being intricately connected, founded on complex relationships. In addition, the researcher is seen as a critical link in inquiry rather than as a distant "knower" who seeks to accomplish the "known." The role of the researcher is recognized and valued; the persons being studied are seen as having (or at least deserving) a hand in shaping the research.

The idea of relationships and connectedness presents a direct contrast to the tenets of Logical Positivism that advocate reductionism, context and value-free inquiry, and Truth and foundationism. In fact, this conceptualization of science addresses many of the limitations and criticisms of strict empiricism particularly Logical Positivism. It also, however, raises several concerns about science and the effectiveness of a proposed "feminist" view. First, such ideas of connectedness and relationships among elements in the world are legitimate questions that could be levied in response to Logical Positivism. It is not clear, however, that these are inherently gendered ideas. Gilligan (1982) astutely points out this in the introduction to her often-cited text:

> The different voice I describe is characterized not by gender but by theme. Its association with women is an empirical observation, and it is primarily through women's voices that I trace its development. But this association is not absolute, and the contrasts between male and female voices are presented here to highlight a distinction between two modes of thought and to focus a problem of interpretation rather than to represent a generalization about either sex. (p. 2)

Gilligan describes her interest as being primarily in the "interaction of experience and thought, in different voices and the dialogues to which they give rise" (p. 2). Feminists undoubtedly will claim that women's experiences as a direct result of gender will affect the interaction and the resulting dialogues. There is reason to be cautious about over-generalizing such a position, a point that Harding (1986) makes clear in her discussion of fractured identities.

---

[1]Dr. McClintock's incredible accomplishments deserve more than a passing reference. McClintock received her PhD in botany from Cornell University in 1927. At the time, women scientists were rare enough, and women were not permitted to major in genetics at Cornell. She studied the genetic composition of maize and is credited with numerous groundbreaking discoveries particularly the idea of the transposable nature of genes. McClintock shows the impermanence of many "facts" and emphasizes the need to look at an entire organism to understand its nature. McClintock was the third woman elected to the National Academy of Sciences, a recipient of the National Medal of Science, the first recipient of a MacArthur Foundation grant, and the first woman to be sole recipient of the Nobel Prize in Physiology or Medicine. See E. F. Keller's (1983b) biography for additional information. The National Library of Medicine profiles of science is available on the NLM web site as an additional interesting source (http://profiles.nlm.nih.gov/).

A similar concern is related to the labeling of particular views of science and of reality as reflective of a particular gender. Feminists argue that science is necessarily gendered and that traditional empirical modes of inquiry reflect an androcentric view. The influence of the "knower" on what is "known" seems fairly obvious, and there is sound reason to question the possibility of complete objectivity. The observation that such science is necessarily male is more troublesome. Men historically have occupied the majority of positions as scientists and continue to dominate many fields in the traditional sciences. Logical Positivism, commonly associated with traditional science, also has significant limitations as noted earlier. These limitations are legitimate points of criticism without reference to gender, however, and applying the label of gender can have the simultaneous effect of distracting while strengthening the central points of the critique.

IMPLICATIONS FOR NURSING

Peggy Chinn (1989), a noted nurse expert in theory development, acknowledges the potential contradiction embodied in references to gender in association with knowledge development, and offers a more comprehensive view of knowledge. She sees nursing as being strongly focused on "wholeness" as a core element of health. Building on Carper's (1978) patterns of knowing, Chinn points out that nurses:

> see the world through a lens of integration and wholeness. We cannot conceive of knowing in any partial way as sufficient. We cannot rely on any one way of knowing that disregards another dimension of experience. We know we experience reality in a whole way. (p. 72)

Chinn dreamed of a nursing construction of the world with peace and health at the center of all activity, with nurses creating "environments that comfort and heal" (p. 73). Nurses would be person-focused, understanding, and developing compassion of the experiences of all others.

While such a development is possible without feminism, Chinn (1989) argues that "feminist thinking brings another dimension to the possibilities we can envision for the future" (p. 73). This dimension provides insights into power relationships and the distribution of power and freedom throughout the population. This idea of power has a definite political component, which is appropriate in that "every aspect of our personal circumstances as women, and as nurses, grows out of, and creates, larger political realities in the world" (p. 73). Feminism attempts to point out that personal problems and situations, such as the working conditions and scope of practice of nurses, have a political component; treating problems only on a personal level, as if they were the problems of the individual rather than the context, allows the political dynamics to persist. Thus, what is immediately personal also must be regarded as political (p. 73); change needs to address the context and political situation and not be limited to the individual.

Political activism on the part of women has been an important part of U.S. and international history. The alliance between feminism as a political movement and nursing has not been a natural one. Historically men have had strong roots in nursing with nursing services offered through military and religious venues often being provided by males (Bunting & Campbell, 1990). Over time, nursing shifted to become a female dominated vocation. Attempts to organize to promote the professional status of nursing resulted in some alliances between nurses and philanthropic women invested in social reforms (Bunting & Campbell, 1990; Kalisch & Kalisch, 1995). Nurses worked to establish their own support mechanisms and to develop their own professional identity. This role in promoting nursing as a profession was not seen as being closely linked to promoting the status of women. The American Nurses Association, for example, did not officially support the right for women to vote in the early years after the organization's founding. Nurses, thus, contributed to some of the distance between feminism and nursing.

The women's movement in later years also may have alienated some nurses for maintaining traditionally women's work roles in a time of role redefinition and advocacy for expanded opportunities for women. Some women have rejected the radicalism of select elements in the women's movement as well. In the 1970s and 1980s, however, any lines of division seem to have become blurred and at least some agreement is evident on central issues. The way in which gender affects issues related to nurses' work and the steps needed to improve nurses' situations are likely to continue to be the focus of much debate for years to come.

As noted previously, the combination of the personal with the political in feminist philosophy is relevant to the work of nurses and reflects a central feature of postmodernism that is exemplified particularly well in feminism. The postmodern ideas of multiple realities, social construction of experiences, and alternate conceptions of truth also are evident in feminist philosophy. Ideas of marginalization and power are consistently present whenever gender enters into discussion. Feminism reflects many major issues confronting the development of a knowledge base for nursing in a contemporary context.

 ## CONCLUSION

These key issues associated with postmodernism and particularly feminism are summarized well by Patty Lather (1991) when she identifies the assumptions for her own work. These include the limitations or "failure" of traditional science (i.e., positivism), the influence of values on science, the potential contributions of critical approaches, and the need to empower persons "to change as well as understand the world" (p. 3). She agrees with other writers of this genre (Derrida, 1974; Lattas, 1989) that postmodernism is not the next step in philosophical development, consequently a "successor regime," but a mixed compilation of "often contradictory ideas and practices" generally referred to as "postmodern" (p. 5).

In this sense, feminism stands as a philosophical view that is still emerging and evolving as a tradition. It has received considerable attention in nursing as a way to capture the experiences of women as recipients of care. Simultaneously it compels nurses to reflect on their own positions as care providers, power-holders, and their roles within the broader health system and society. Further development of the philosophy and related modes of inquiry in the area of feminism is likely to continue for some time.

 # FOR DISCUSSION

1. Discuss the basic ontologic position that underlies feminist approaches to knowledge development.
2. For a selected phenomenon of interest in nursing, discuss how viewpoints would vary according to feminist empiricism, feminist standpoint theory, and feminist postmodernism.
3. Discuss similarities and differences between feminist philosophy in general and the major tenets of postmodern philosophy
4. Discuss strengths and limitations of feminist approaches to inquiry in the development of nursing knowledge.
5. The traditional criteria for evaluating empirical research are not consistent with the philosophy of feminism. Describe criteria that would be appropriate for evaluating the contributions of feminist inquiry in the development of nursing knowledge.

REFERENCES

Allen, D. G. (1992). Feminism, relativism, and the philosophy of science: An overview. In J. L. Thompson, D. G. Allen, & L. Rodrigues-Fisher (Eds.), *Critique, resistance, and action: Working papers in the politics of nursing* (Publ. No. 14-2504, pp. 1–19). New York: National League for Nursing Press.

Belenky, M. F., Clinchy, B. M., Goldberger, N. R., & Tarule, J. M. (1986). *Women's ways of knowing: The development of self, voice, and mind.* US: Basic Books.

Bunting, S., & Campbell, J. C. (1990). Feminism and nursing: Historical perspectives. *Advances in Nursing Science, 12*(4), 11–24.

Carper, B. A. (1978). Fundamental patterns of knowing in nursing. *Advances in Nursing Science, 1*(1), 13–23.

Carson, R. (1941). *Under the sea-wind, a naturalist's picture of ocean life.* New York: Simon and Schuster.

Carson, R. (1962). *Silent spring.* Boston: Houghton Mifflin.

Chinn, P. L. (1989). Nursing patterns of knowing and feminist thought. *Nursing and Health Care, 10,* 71–75.

Derrida, J. (1974). *Of grammatology* (G. C. Spivak, Trans.). Baltimore: Johns Hopkins University Press.

Gilligan, C. (1982). *In a different voice: Psychological theory and women's development.* Cambridge, MA: Harvard University Press.

Harding, S. (1986). *The science question in feminism.* Ithaca, NY: Cornell University.

Harding, S. (1991). *Whose science? Whose knowledge?* Ithaca, NY: Cornell University.

Kalisch, P. A., & Kalisch, B. J. (1995). *The advance of American nursing*. Philadelphia: J. B. Lippincott.

Keller, E. F. (1983a). Gender and science. In S. Harding & M. B. Hintikka (Eds.), *Discovering reality*, (pp. 187–205). Boston: D. Reidel.

Keller, E. F. (1983b). *A feeling for the organism: The life and work of Barbara McClintock*. New York: W. H. Freeman.

Kohlberg, L. (1981). *Essays on moral development*. San Francisco: Harper & Row.

Lather, P. (1991). *Getting smart: Feminist research and pedagogy with/in the postmodern*. New York: Routledge.

Lattas, J. (1989). Feminism as a proper name. *Australian Feminist Studies, 9*, 85–96.

Power, F. C., Higgins-D'Alessandro, A., & Kohlberg, L. (1989). *Lawrence Kohlberg's approach to moral education*. New York: Columbia University Press.

Smithsonian Institution. The Seneca Falls convention. Available online at http://www.npg.si.edu/col/Seneca/senfalls1.htm. (Accessed October 28, 2003) .

Stanton, E. C. (1889). *A history of woman suffrage* (Vol. 1). Rochester, NY: Fowler and Wells.

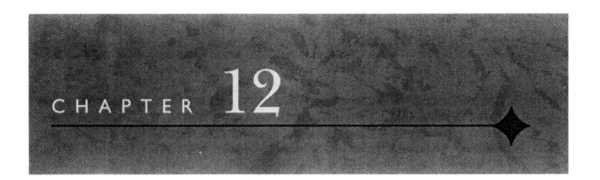

CHAPTER 12

Problems and Practicalities in Developing Nursing Knowledge

The history of nursing knowledge development shows a progressive effort to understand the complex nature of the discipline and to strengthen the philosophical grounding for inquiry and further development. Topics emphasized in this quest include the nature of "science," the relationship between "science" and "knowledge," the ideas of truth and theory, and, more recently, the notion of "evidence." Because of the lack of any definitive answers to the philosophical questions relevant in nursing, it would be both reasonable and practical to consider this ongoing exploration as endless. As a result, nurses must continue to stay connected with philosophical and social changes and avoid complacency as they continually seek better ways of approaching nursing knowledge.

Nursing and philosophy literature provides numerous ideas about ways to develop knowledge. Some ideas include the development of formal theories that can be expressed in propositional forms (Ayer, 1959; see also the writings of Carnap, 1967; Hempel, 1952; Schlick, 1974, 1979); the acquisition of sensory data to establish "Truth" (Locke, 1690/1975) or, according to Popper (1976, 1979), less falsehood; the clarification of paradigms (Kuhn, 1962, 1970, 1977) or research traditions (Laudan, 1977); development of a coherent and useful conceptual repertoire (Toulmin, 1972); or enlightenment, deconstruction, or "emancipation" from power, authority, and other social and cultural constructions that shape or give meaning to human existence (Bowers & Moore, 1997; Gadamer, 1975, 1976; Habermas, 1968; Harden, 2000; Harding, 1991; Horkheimer & Adorno, 1972). Philosophers and nurse scholars have argued that these and other aims are the proper goal of knowledge development efforts.

Each of these objectives has some strengths and weaknesses. In addition to assessing strengths, however, it also is important to consider the "fit" with nursing, in other words, how consistent a view is with the goals and nature of nursing. Other concerns include what might be considered descriptive and prescriptive credibility. The term **descriptive credibility** here refers to the extent to which a philosophical position reflects or describes the way scholars in a discipline pursue knowledge and expansion of the discipline. **Prescriptive credibility** is applied here in regard to whether or not a viewpoint presents a meaningful or defensible position on how knowledge should be developed in the future (Box 12-1).

ENSURING A "FIT" AMONG KNOWLEDGE AND NURSING GOALS

Awareness of the nature of nursing obviously is a central focus of such considerations. Nurse scholars need to avoid the substantial pitfalls associated with merely following emerging trends. While it is important to be aware of changes in philosophy and in social and health care contexts, it is equally important to maintain a critical eye in evaluating new ideologies. Ideological changes need to be considered in regard to their fit with nurses' knowledge and roles and the potential to contribute to development of the knowledge base. Forms of inquiry as well as disciplinary changes that are considered for adoption need to be reviewed for their appropriateness to nursing's role and objectives and not merely because they are currently fashionable.

A clear sense of the focus, values, and identity of the discipline of nursing, therefore, is very helpful in evaluating ideas for their appropriateness to nursing knowledge development. Nursing inquiry starts with awareness of existing beliefs and ideology about the phenomena being investigated and the potential contributions of the investigation to knowledge development. Understanding the current position is essential to determining the direction to be pursued next. This is not to be interpreted as a second wave of the argument about "borrowed" versus "unique" knowledge, such that nurses should focus only on developing "nursing" knowledge, while other forms would reflect the focus of other disciplines and thus seem to be "borrowed." There is no ownership of knowledge; in fact, one challenge of current

---

BOX 12-1

DESCRIPTIVE AND PRESCRIPTIVE CREDIBILITY

Prescriptive and descriptive credibility can be used to evaluate the appropriateness of a philosophical position. For prescriptive credibility, the central question is, "Does the view present an appropriate guide for action and for progress in the field?" For descriptive credibility, the assumption is that some existing knowledge development activity works, and the viewpoint should reflect what is happening, in other words, it should adequately describe the activities. A position that does not fit with existing knowledge development activities might be missing key components or otherwise lacking in usefulness.

---

inquiry is to create more inclusive contexts to allow widespread dissemination and collaboration to broaden perspectives represented in inquiry. Nurses do need to ensure, however, that current work enhances the knowledge base of nursing. There is much that needs to be uncovered, explored, and developed in nursing. The contributions of nurses to human health and social improvement are outstanding throughout history. This legacy needs to be revised as contexts and needs change and new knowledge created to enhance these changing roles. While nurses should not be discouraged from pursuing research of direct benefit to nurses regardless of fit, there does need to be continuing attention to what is most needed in the discipline. Without such attention, pressing needs in the discipline might not be addressed; nurses who need the knowledge in their own practice or inquiry may not find the resources they need to substantiate their work.

It is tempting to adopt a perspective of **pluralism** in which a variety of approaches to inquiry are considered acceptable. That is perhaps the most open and inclusive approach; a number of authors have advocated having an array of methods from which to choose or possibly to combine methods as appropriate to a particular study (Baker, Norton, Young, & Ward, 1998; Coward, 1990; Letourneau & Allen, 1999). Combining approaches or even choosing from a variety does present some challenges. From a philosophical standpoint, the various traditions available for consideration are philosophically incongruent and cannot simply be combined or even compared to the others. Each presents a different ontology and uses different language and criteria for judging quality. This inability to compare views directly is known as the problem of **incommensurability**. Products of different philosophies or paradigms, particularly theories, are incommensurable, which means that they cannot be compared directly. Instead they must be viewed from the standpoint of the values and orientation that underlie their development. The difficulty in making comparisons applies to philosophical traditions as well because each tradition is based on a different world view with its own goals and criteria for evaluating quality and progress.

Feyerabend (1975), an Austrian philosopher of the mid-20th century, advocated for maximum creativity and innovation in knowledge development. He denounced any attempt to prescribe a single method for science, promoting instead the ideology that "anything goes." This statement likely has some immediate appeal especially having explored the confusing array of possibilities for knowledge development presented in the history of Western philosophy. Creativity and freedom to explore new areas and methodologies are critical to discovery and continuing progress and innovation. Yet this presents a similar problem in regard to evaluating outcomes of knowledge development or "scientific" work. Multiplism, pluralism, "anything goes," and other potential views and approaches to knowledge development require that some criteria be considered to evaluate their individual contributions. Resources to support inquiry and means for dissemination are not without limits nor are the time and energy of investigators and scholars limitless. Ultimately decisions must be made about the best use of such resources, what are fruitful and potentially productive areas and modes of inquiry, and what avenues are likely to yield results meaningful to the discipline and helpful to moving it in the desired direction.

A practical approach to this situation is to look at the discipline's needs and goals and use those as a guide for decision making. The nature of nursing seems to dictate that knowledge development activities be useful and capable of application in the work of nurses. That work is quite diverse, however, allowing for the possibility of multiple foci and directions for research. That diversity also raises the question of how such variability can be accommodated while still maintaining some integrity, or some common identity, in the discipline as "nursing."

Practicality sometimes invokes the idea of **pragmatism** and the terms may be used interchangeably in everyday conversation. In philosophy, pragmatism has a specific meaning and refers to a school of philosophy. The American philosopher, William James, often is credited with being the founder of Pragmatism as a school in philosophy. James (1907) describes the "pragmatic method" in the following way after recounting a heated debate among his colleagues about the nature of the actions of a squirrel circling around a tree:

> I tell this trivial anecdote because it is a peculiarly simple example of what I wish now to speak of as the pragmatic method. The pragmatic method is primarily a method of settling metaphysical disputes that otherwise might be interminable. Is the world one or many? Fated or free? Material or spiritual? These are notions that may or may not hold good of the world, and disputes over such notions are unending. The pragmatic method in such cases is to try to interpret each notion by tracing its respective practical consequences. What difference would it practically make to any one if this notion rather than that notion were true? If no practical difference whatever can be traced, then the alternatives mean practically the same thing, and all dispute is idle. Whenever a dispute is serious, we ought to be able to show some practical difference that must follow from one side or the other's being right. (p. 42–43)

Pragmatism, in simple terms, is focused on the practical consequences of various possibilities: What difference would it make if one statement were true in comparison to another? This does bear some similarity to the idea of being practical, yet the philosophy of pragmatism is not limited to examining tangible outcomes as consequences of beliefs.

TAKING A "PROBLEM-SOLVING" APPROACH

A philosophy of **problem solving** is closely related to the nurses' need to have knowledge development activities that are applicable and relevant to the science and work of nurses. One variation of a problem-solving approach was presented by Laudan (1977; see Chapter 7), who argued that the idea of problem solving "is more a cliché than a philosophy" (p. 11). It is possible that his comment was derived from a lack of emphasis on solving problems and the general outcomes of scientific work. Much of the philosophy of science has been concerned with the theoretical products (Logical Positivism) or the structures and processes of science and scientific decision making (Historicism). Science, in fact, involves a combination of credible work with meaningful outcomes. A comprehensive philosophical base that recognizes these contributions and that ties scientific work to the knowledge base of a discipline would seem to be a good fit and a productive approach for nursing knowledge development.

Kuhn (1962, 1970) also presented an early form of this idea of problem solving; he used the phrase "puzzle-solving," however, to describe the intellectual processes that characterize scientific activity. Kuhn was reacting to the emphasis of the Logical Positivists on the product of scientific activity, specifically the development of theory, and he called attention instead to the processes of science. Laudan (1977) similarly emphasized a solution-focused approach and referred to science as "essentially a problem-solving activity" (p. 11). For both philosophers, the focus of science is not on generating products that look a certain way but on the merits of the work in solving problems relevant to the discipline.

Toulmin (1972) added further emphasis to the problem-solving possibilities of science by giving attention to the gap between the needs of a discipline and its existing knowledge and capabilities (see Chapter 8). According to Toulmin, a problem can be associated with any need of the discipline. According to this view, a problem for nursing can involve anything that nurses need to understand and for which they currently lack the knowledge and capabilities. Laudan argued that it was sufficient for a situation merely to be thought a problem; no specific criteria or documentation were necessary.

In this view, problems are basically epistemic in nature and should not be confused with practice problems or problems of implementation. Because this problem-solving work focuses on the development of knowledge, the discipline's needs for additional knowledge should be a primary consideration in the definition of problems. Inquiry to answer questions about whether or not nurses should be required to work mandatory overtime is not likely to contribute to expanding the epistemic base of the discipline. The conceptualization of quality (in regard to care), however, is a significant and enduring concern in nursing. Inquiry to clarify, delineate, or otherwise expand understanding of quality would contribute substantively to nursing's knowledge base and might reveal that the length of the nurse's work day is an appropriate concern. The inquiry may look quite similar but there is a considerable difference because work on mandatory overtime as a sole focus does not have a direct link to the knowledge base of the discipline; inquiry into quality and the possibility of a relationship with overtime work by nurses does draw on a disciplinary focus. While this may seem a minor point, the potential for building a knowledge base organized to meet the discipline's focus and needs could be greater when inquiry is based on a disciplinary orientation.

Changes in research methods over time comprise another example of a problem for the discipline. Qualitative methods have been articulated with greater clarity and specificity over the last several decades. Much of the work to enhance such methods has been stimulated by the need of nurses and scholars in other disciplines to devise credible ways to capture individual experiences and the impact of situations on human beings' lives. Recognition of the limitations of controlled and presumably objective approaches to inquiry also created a need for ways to address problems that were not amenable to such approaches or that could not be understood adequately using traditional methods. Statistically-oriented research is changing as well with greater emphasis currently on uncovering complex relationships among phenomena rather than merely testing discrete hypotheses.

This situation with the evolution of research methods points out particularly well how problem identification and definition can change as the needs of the discipline and the challenges faced change over time. In nursing, pronounced changes have occurred in human health conditions, social contexts, and environmental states; all these affect the problems identified as appropriate for emphasis within a discipline. Political influences also can be exceptionally strong because these promote or discourage inquiry in certain areas by making resources available to promote only certain types and foci for investigation. Political influences are not limited to governmental areas or sources typically identified as "political." Disciplines generally have their own influences through reward systems and often provide resources through grants and awards. Disciplines also create and control opportunities for dissemination and other means for exchange of ideas (Laudan, 1977, 1984; Toulmin, 1972). Nursing problems also should be expected to mirror major trends in society and health care in general. Various mechanisms, particularly in regard to sharing information and funding sources, can interfere with a fit between the needs of the greater society and the priorities set by the discipline.

Consistent with the epistemic rather than the purely functional nature of problems, there needs to be an emphasis on "knowing" rather than "doing." Correcting an existing situation may be of immediate practical benefit; in a field such as nursing, that can be a significant and meaningful accomplishment. But a problem in the sense discussed here cannot be considered solved until members of the discipline understand how the outcome was accomplished. Without such understanding, it is difficult to have the necessary knowledge of the mechanisms at work in the situation to have confidence in how the results were achieved. Examples can be found throughout the history of health care such as in Nightingale's (1860/1969) work on clean environments, Semmelweis' examination of childbirth fever, and recent discoveries about the origins of gastric ulcers and the link between dietary fats and heart disease. None of these situations were accepted as solutions to problems until the mechanisms of action were understood. Sometimes the underlying mechanisms are demonstrated by scientists other than the one who generated the original idea (Box 12-2). History also shows how problems change over time in response to new knowledge and changes in context. Some of these changes can be seen in the path from the ancient humoral theory of illness through an increased understanding of anatomy (such as Galen, Harvey, and Boyle contributed; see Boyle, 1979; Brock, 1972; Galen, 1997; Harvey, 1958) via the creation of the microscope and the advent of "germ" theory to more recent biochemical and genetic foci in health and illness.

Forms of Nursing Problems

The problems confronted in developing the knowledge base of nursing exist in many forms. Empirical problems are likely to be most familiar to nurses and involve aspects of physical reality in need of exploration. Empirical problems involve elements that can be experienced through the senses; physiologic phenomena such as laboratory values, vital signs, and wound healing measures provide particularly clear examples of such problems in nursing.

Conceptual problems also are very relevant in the process of developing the knowledge base of the discipline. Conceptual problems have received far less attention than empirical problems as a focus of inquiry for many reasons. The emphasis in science, derived partly from Logical Positivism, has been on physical reality. This focus served to relegate nonempirical aspects of reality to the realm of the meaningless or nonsensical. Recognizing a legitimate role for concepts and conceptual problems would allow a human cognitive element to enter the approach to the physical world. Concepts, after all, are mental constructions; the introduction of a human element inherent in any reference to concepts would

BOX 12-2

PROBLEM-SOLVING EXAMPLE

Pasteur showed a bacteriologic basis for Semmelweis' recommended aseptic techniques, converting Semmelweis' accomplishments from what Kuhn would have referred to as an anomaly into a solved problem.

seem counter to the desired objective nature of science. Concepts have been regarded in traditional science merely as words or names for phenomena rather than worthy of exploration. An extensive volume of literature on concepts, however, shows that this is an inadequate view of the nature and importance of these cognitive tools. Clearly the value and significance of how things are conceptualized does have a place in the development of knowledge. Further, many of science's most pressing problems arise from how things are conceptualized rather than how they are observed empirically.

More contemporary views of science vary from allowing conceptual problems as an important focus of inquiry (Laudan, 1977) to possibly acknowledging that all science is conceptual in nature. In his discussion of understanding as primarily a process of concept development, Toulmin (1972) leans in the direction of all science as conceptual in nature. Rodgers and Knafl (2000) also demonstrate the dominant role of concepts in the development of knowledge. Regardless of the value placed on concepts, it is clear that conceptual problems need to be given an important status in advancing the knowledge base of the discipline.

Relevance of a Problem-Solving Approach to Knowledge

A problem-solving approach to knowledge development has many advantages for nursing. A strength of this approach, which may seem rather obvious, is that a problem-solving focus has immediate practical application. There is an overwhelming need for relevant and applicable knowledge in nursing; consequently "solving problems" would seem particularly appealing as a focus of inquiry. As noted before, however, problem solving as a philosophy involves an epistemic focus, not merely the ability to "fix" a currently troublesome situation in the discipline. An accurate interpretation of this position indicates that a problem cannot be confronted effectively unless there is full understanding of the knowledge base underlying the troublesome situation. Relief of discomfort, promotion of health, and cure of disease alone do not contribute to the discipline's future progress and growth unless there is some understanding of how or why the outcome was achieved.

A problem-solving approach is consistent with both the knowledge-oriented and the practice-oriented goals of nursing. Laudan (1977) and Toulmin (1972) also emphasize the dynamic and changing nature of problems. This is consistent with the value system of nursing, which views individuals as diverse and changing and their individual realities also as constantly subject to change (Donaldson & Crowley, 1978; Flaskerud & Halloran, 1980; Schultz, 1987). Nursing, therefore, needs an approach to knowledge development that allows or ideally promotes flexibility and innovation. In that regard, a problem-solving approach has significant potential to contribute to the discipline's progress through understanding how to achieve desired outcomes and an action's effectiveness.

A "problem-solving" approach to knowledge is compatible with a nursing perspective and with the need for the nurses' knowledge base to remain relevant as contexts change. It also is consistent with the many different needs in the discipline. Maintaining an emphasis on selected theories or specific concepts or phenomena that might have seemed acceptable in the past places inappropriate limits on the work to expand the knowledge base. A focus on problem solving instead enables work to proceed in multiple areas at the same time and allows for the possibility of collaborative work. In a problem-solving perspective, it is reasonable to pursue work to develop taxonomies and to develop outcome criteria and quality assurance measures while simultaneously focusing on the individual narratives or subjective experiences of the patients or clients with whom nurses work.

This approach might seem a bit too open or flexible for those accustomed to more specific or restrictive approaches to "science." In such contexts, it might lack the specificity and the rigid criteria that typically accompany "science." The current state of nursing, however, mandates such openness and flexibility in knowledge development efforts. Problems for nursing inquiry exist in a wide variety of forms including the need for classification systems consistent with technological innovation, the need for broader understanding of empirical phenomena, and also the need for greater understanding of individual situations and how people experience and interpret health and illness situations. Rather than being perceived as too loose or lacking prescriptive focus, a problem-solving approach enables the creativity and innovation appropriate to address a varying and constantly changing array of problems.

In discussing directions for nursing theory development in the 21st century, Meleis (1992) described some of the characteristics of nursing as a discipline. She pointed out that

> knowing results from careful systematic research or from repeated experiences in clinical practice. By reflecting on knowledge from these sources and interpreting the meanings of relationships experienced by all parties concerned, and by pulling what is known in the context of feelings, values, and different perspectives, better understanding can be achieved. (p. 113)

Nurses must be encouraged to think broadly in identifying new problems for inquiry. Nurse scholars have made significant strides while utilizing disparate biomedical, psychological, and sociological approaches to health situations. Integration among these various elements still needs to be enhanced with additional focus on the complex interactions that occur among aspects of human existence.

Success in solving problems in the discipline, therefore, depends on the ability to see situations from new perspectives, to identify problems appropriately, and to apply various forms of inquiry effectively. There must be support for developing new forms of inquiry as well because different problems and challenges may exceed the limits of established methods. Addressing the discipline's problems also requires understanding the discipline itself in order to define problems in a manner consistent with the discipline's "intellectual ideals."

This disciplinary focus may be one of the most significant yet perhaps the least obvious contributions of the problem-solving approach to the development of nursing. The context in which research occurs, particularly in regard to political and social influences, easily can influence nurse scientists to view problems using criteria driven to some extent by available resources and professional expectations and aspirations. The result can be that contextual factors, particularly those external to the discipline, drive the development of nursing. A keen awareness of the goals, values, and contributions of nursing to the health of people and their environments is essential to progress in the discipline.

Problem solving, as described by both Laudan (1977) and Toulmin (1972), involves a clear human component consistent with historicist and postmodern ideologies. The judgments and values of the discipline and the individual researchers have an important role in knowledge development. This aspect of the approach poses a stark contrast with positivist philosophies that advocate (and assume to be possible) a value-free and objective approach emphasizing "science."

Problem solving avoids the pitfalls of a distinction between science and knowledge. It also enables a connection between the practical and the philosophical as well as the opportunity for inquiry focused on meaningful knowledge development. Scholars can be encouraged to pursue passions connected to useful outcomes. Awareness of both the application and the discipline's intellectual goals can ensure continued development relevant both to nursing and the people and their situations addressed through nursing inquiry. Such an approach can be promoted by stimulating creative ideas and perspectives for purposes of both problem identification and effective inquiry to advance the knowledge base.

The Role of Existing Research in Problem Solving

The problem-solving approach calls for the identification of problems relevant to the discipline and the pursuit of inquiry to resolve these deficits in current knowledge. Problem solving provides a way not only to identify areas for future research to ensure progress in the discipline but also a way to organize and interpret existing knowledge and information. In nursing, many actions have been based on tradition or anecdotal reports. An early attempt to improve this situation called for research utilization to ensure that research results were implemented in practice to bring nursing practice in line with current knowledge. The research utilization movement was stimulated by recognition that considerable research existed to address significant nursing concerns, yet in many cases, results were not used to change nursing practice.

An extensive amount of research has been conducted to explore issues associated with research utilization. A particularly strong effort has been devoted to exploring factors that promote or impede the application of research results in clinical settings (Funk, Tornquist, & Champagne, 1995). By the early 1990s, three distinct models had evolved to promote the utilization of research results to improve nursing care delivery (White, Leske, & Pearcy, 1995). The CURN (Brett, 1987; Larson, 1989), Stetler (1985, 2001), and Iowa (Titler & Mentes,

1999) models all presented various ways to conceptualize the "gap" between research and practice and to promote changes in practice based on application of research results. The results of this effort included research-based protocols and practice guidelines, organizational change to facilitate application of research in practice settings, and efforts to raise awareness and increase research utilization skills of nurses in clinical settings such as educational programs, links with academic research centers, research facilitator arrangements, research committees and journal clubs. Improving the quality of care was an obvious focus in this effort.

The research utilization effort also was growing in other aspects of health care during the 1980s and 1990s. Research utilization has evolved to be known throughout health care as **Evidence Based Practice** (EBP). In 1997, the United States Agency for Health Care Policy and Research (now the Agency for Healthcare Research and Quality [AHRQ]) accelerated the effort to bring research findings into health care practice by establishing a number of Evidence-based Practice Centers (EPCs). The purpose of the EPCs is to "develop evidence reports and technology assessments based on rigorous, comprehensive synthesis and analyses of the scientific literature on topics relevant to clinical, social science/behavioral, economic, and other health care organization and delivery issues" (AHRQ, accessed 1/14/04). Evidence-based practice has become a focus in many countries as well as an underlying principle of emerging models of education. Evidence-based medicine has been described as a "new paradigm" for medical education and practice. In contrast to a specific focus on "research" as with "research utilization," an evidence-based approach requires use of data or other forms of "evidence" in making decisions about appropriate interventions. It does not mandate, however, that the data be collected through systematic investigations or other formal means. (Evidence-Based Medicine Working Group, 1992). Standards of rigor including peer review always are desirable. The intent of evidence-based practice is to avoid the obvious pitfalls of allowing tradition, anecdote, and authority to guide care delivery and to establish some sort of credible support for actions.

Ingersoll (2000) uses the terms "evidence-based nursing" in regard to the application of this approach to nursing care delivery. She describes a number of concerns about EBP for nurses, however, including limited mention of the use of qualitative research results in the literature of EBP. Other concerns have been associated with the lack of connection between theory and practice and the need for consideration of the ethical implications of interventions (Ingersoll, 2000; Upton, 1999). Ingersoll suggests a definition of EBP that maintains the current emphasis on systematic review of published research but also reflects the importance of theory-based action appropriate to an individual situation and needs (p. 152). Evidence-based nursing will continue to be a subject of debate for some time while issues about the nature of evidence, criteria for evaluating quality of evidence, and links between evidence and a knowledge or philosophical base in nursing are explored further (Romyn et al., 2003)

CONCLUSION

Nurse researchers have long sought to connect "science" and "practice." The attempt to do so gained considerable impetus with the research utilization and EBP developments. These efforts do a great deal to stimulate the application of research results in nursing care situations. The application of research results not only improves practice presumably by providing a credible basis for care decisions but also similarly renders the research more useful. Research results that are read and used only by other researchers are of little benefit to those expected to act in accordance with the discipline's knowledge base.

The need for a relationship between research and application of results is nearly self-evident. To be defensible and especially to have a greater likelihood of being effective, practice must be based on something other than authority or tradition. However, a link to the discipline's knowledge base is missing from this equation. Nursing practice does not always reflect existing knowledge. As just discussed, one explanation for this situation is the failure to apply research results in practice. Another cause, however, is the lack of a connection between the epistemic and ontologic positions espoused in the discipline and the theoretical basis for nursing and the actions taken by nurses. In other words, many activities in which nurses engage may not reflect the nurses' knowledge base. The engagement of nurses in "non-nursing" tasks is well known throughout the profession. The concern here in discussion of the activities of nurses is not about nurses doing things that do not require preparation as a nurse but nurses thinking with the perspective and the awareness of the knowledge base that reflects the commitment, values, and world view espoused in nursing.

A problem-solving approach to knowledge is compatible with closing the gap between research, practice, and development of the discipline. Knowledge needs to be tied not only to the needs of those who apply the knowledge but also to the growth of the knowledge base in general. The discipline's continuing growth and progress can benefit from recognition of how addressing problems through research promotes progress for the discipline as a whole.

Problem solving has the potential to provide a means for linking these aspects of nursing. Unlike philosophies that dictate a specific product of science, problem solving places more emphasis on why particular studies or forms of inquiry may be pursued and how the results contribute important knowledge. There has been reason for caution throughout this text, however, about adopting any one approach without diligent consideration of the strengths, limitations, and fit with nursing's goals and needs. That caveat continues to apply in regard to problem solving. This approach offers an alternative to reliance on specific methodologies, discrete conceptual repertoires, a limited array of phenomena, or other approaches to delineating nursing knowledge development. Problem solving may be of value in directing knowledge development effort in a manner that not only contributes needed information for nurses who must apply the knowledge but also work that will benefit and expand the discipline and the intellectual base of nursing.

FOR DISCUSSION

1. Discuss how a problem-solving approach is congruent with the goals and perspective of nursing.
2. Identify and discuss one empirical problem and one conceptual problem relevant to the development of the knowledge base in nursing.
3. Discuss how a problem-solving approach to knowledge development is both similar to and distinct from evidence-based practice.
4. Discuss strengths and limitations of a problem-solving approach to knowledge development.

REFERENCES

Agency for Healthcare Research and Quality. *Evidence based practice centers: Synthesizing scientific evidence to improve quality and effectiveness in health care.* Available online http://www.ahcpr.gov/clinic/epc. (Accessed January 14, 2004).

Ayer, A. J. (Ed.). (1959). *Logical positivism.* New York: Free Press.

Baker, C., Norton, S., Young, P., & Ward, S. (1998). An exploration of methodological pluralism in nursing research. *Research in Nursing and Health, 21,* 545–555.

Bowers, R., & Moore, K. N. (1997). Bakhtin, nursing narratives, and dialogical consciousness. *Advances in Nursing Science, 19*(3), 70–77.

Brett, J. L. (1987). Use of nursing practice research findings. *Nursing Research, 36,* 344–349.

Brock, A. J. (Ed. & Trans.). (1972). *Greek medicine, being extracts illustrative of medical writers from Hippocrates to Galen.* London: Dent.

Carnap, R. (1967). *The logical structure of the world: Pseudoproblems in philosophy.* (R. A. George, Trans.). Berkeley: University of California Press.

Coward, D. D. (1990). Critical multiplism: A research strategy for nursing science. *Image: Journal of Nursing Scholarship, 22,* 163–167.

Donaldson, S. K., & Crowley, D. M. (1978). The discipline of nursing. *Nursing Outlook, 26,* 113–120.

Evidence-Based Medicine Working Group. (1992). Evidence-based medicine: A new approach to teaching the practice of medicine. *Journal of the American Medical Association, 268,* 2420–2425.

Feyerabend, P. K. (1975). *Against method.* London: Humanities Press.

Flaskerud, J. H., & Halloran, E. J. (1980). Areas of agreement in nursing theory development. *Advances in Nursing Science, 3*(1), 1–7.

Funk, S. G., Tornquist, E. M., & Champagne, M. T. (1995). Barriers and facilitators of research utilization: An integrative review. *Nursing Clinics of North America, 30,* 395–407.

Gadamer, H. (1975). *Truth and method.* (G. Barden and J. Cumming, Trans. and Eds.). New York: Seabury Press.

Gadamer, H. (1976). *Philosophical hermeneutics.* (D. E. Linge, Trans.). Berkeley: University of California Press.

Galen (1997). *Selected works.* (P. N. Singer, Trans.). Oxford: Oxford University Press.

Habermas, J. (1968), *Knowledge and human interests.* (J. J. Shapiro, trans.). Boston: Beacon Press.

Harden, J. (2000). Language, discourse and the chronotope: Applying literary theory to the narratives in health care. *Journal of Advanced Nursing, 31,* 506–512.

Harding, S. (1991). *Whose science? Whose knowledge?* Ithaca, NY: Cornell University.

Harvey, W. (1958). *The circulation of the blood.* (K. J. Franklin, Trans.). Oxford: Blackwell Scientific Publications.

Hempel, C. G. (1952). *Philosophy of natural science.* Englewood Cliffs, NJ: Prentice Hall.

Horkheimer, M., & Adorno, T. W. (1972). *Dialectic of enlightenment* (J. Cumming, Trans.). New York: Herder & Herder.

Ingersoll, G. (2000). Evidence-based nursing: What it is and what it isn't. *Nursing Outlook, 48,* 151–152.

James, W. (1907). *Pragmatism.* Cleveland, OH: World Publishing Company.

Kuhn, T. S. (1962). *The structure of scientific revolutions.* Chicago: University of Chicago Press.

Kuhn, T. S. (1970). *The structure of scientific revolutions* (2nd Ed.). Chicago: University of Chicago Press.

Kuhn, T. S. (1977). *The essential tension.* Chicago: University of Chicago Press.

Larson, E. (1989). Using the CURN project to teach research utilization in a baccalaureate program. *Western Journal of Nursing Research, 11,* 593–599.

Laudan, L. (1977). *Progress and its problems: Towards a theory of scientific growth.* Berkeley: University of California Press.

Laudan, L. (1984). *Science and values: The aims of science and their role in scientific debate.* Berkeley: University of California Press.

Letourneau, N., & Allen, M. (1999). Post-positivistic critical multiplism: A beginning dialogue. *Journal of Advanced Nursing, 30,* 623–630.

Locke, J. (1975). *An essay concerning human understanding* (P. Nidditch, Ed.). Oxford: Oxford University Press. (Original work published 1690).

Meleis, A. I. (1992). Directions for nursing theory development in the 21st century. *Nursing Science Quarterly, 5,* 112–117.

Nightingale, F. (1969). *Notes on nursing: What it is, and what it is not.* New York: Dover. (Original work published 1860).

Popper, K. R. (1976). *Conjectures and refutations.* London: Routledge & Kegan Paul. (Original work published 1963).

Popper, K. R. (1979). *Objective knowledge.* Oxford: Oxford University Press. (Original work published 1972).

Rodgers, B. L., & Knafl, K. A. (2000). *Concept development in nursing: Foundations, techniques, and applications.* Philadelphia: W. B. Saunders.

Romyn, D. M., Allen, M. N., Boschma, G., Duncan, S. M., Edgecomb, N., Jensen, L. A., Ross-Kerr, J. C., Marck, P., Salsali, M., Tourangeau, A. E., & Warnock, F. (2003). The notion of evidence in evidence-based practice. *Journal of Professional Nursing, 19,* 184–188.

Schlick, M. (1974). *General theory of knowledge.* (A. E. Blumberg, Trans.). New York: Springer-Verlag.

Schlick, M. (1979). *Philosophical papers.* (H. L. Mulder & B. F. B. van de Velde-Schlick, Ed.; P. Heath, Trans.). Boston: D. Reider Publishing Company.

Schultz, P. R. (1987). Toward holistic inquiry in nursing: A proposal for synthesis of patterns and methods. *Scholarly Inquiry for Nursing Practice: An International Journal, 1,* 135–146.

Stetler, C. B. (1985). Research utilization: Defining the concept. *Image: Journal of Nursing Scholarship, 17,* 40–44.

Stetler, C. B. (2001). Updating the Stetler Model of research utilization to facilitate evidence-based practice. *Nursing Outlook, 49,* 272–279.

Stewart, M. A. (Ed.). *Selected philosophical papers of R. Boyle.* Manchester, England: Manchester University Press.

Titler, M. G., & Mentes, J. C. (1999). Research utilization in gerontological nursing practice. *Journal of Gerontological Nursing, 25*(6), 6–9.

Toulmin, S. (1972). *Human understanding.* Princeton, NJ: Princeton University Press.

Upton, D. J. (1999). How can we achieve evidence-based practice if we have a theory-practice gap in nursing today? *Journal of Advanced Nursing, 29,* 188–193.

White, J. M., Leske, J. S., & Pearcy, J. M. (1995). Models and processes of research utilization. *Nursing Clinics of North America, 30,* 409–420.

CHAPTER 13

Models for Nursing Knowledge Development

KEY IDEAS

analog model
concept development
conceptual model
descriptive theory
discourse
experience
formal theory
grand theory

metatheory
micro-range theory
middle-range theory
model
narrative
situation-specific theory
story
symbolic model

The phrase "models for nursing knowledge development" will certainly generate a variety of images for nurses. The term "models" is most likely to conjure thoughts of all the theories and conceptual models created to guide nurses in their quest to delineate their discipline and as devices to promote research and effective practice. Use of the term "model" in this chapter bears some similarity to that use in its intention to reflect ways of viewing the world of nursing as a guide for knowledge development. A **model** is an illustration or some representation of ideas. Models exist in a variety of forms (Box 13-1). **Symbolic models** provide an organized illustration of an idea using symbols or other pictorial images to represent elements of the idea. This type of model is familiar to nurses who often see flow charts, diagrams, and similar illustrations showing everything from physiologic functions as basic as the Krebs cycle to neurologic pathways, dermatomes, acupuncture points, and circulatory charts.

The **analog model** is another type commonly used in nursing. The analog model works to provide an explanation through construction of an analogy, or a comparison that shows the similarity between two things. Typically in an analog model, a new or unfamiliar idea is compared to something familiar and more likely to be understood. A common example is the description of the heart's functioning by comparison to a pump.

Conceptual models also are common in nursing. This phrase often is applied to the discipline's theoretical formulations created primarily during the 1970s and 1980s. Conceptual models involve linkages among a variety of concepts as a way to illustrate thinking and to provide a visual reference for nurses to use in practice. The term "conceptual model" was used to describe these constructions because of the rather narrow and rigid idea of what counted as "theory" at the time. Some "models" in nursing lacked the specificity and supporting evidence expected for a "theory" so they were considered to be at a lower level of development. As a result, the term conceptual model rather than "theory" was applied.

In this chapter, the term **model** refers to a heuristic model—a plan, idea, or guide for inquiry. The possibilities for models that can promote nursing knowledge development represent an array of ideological, philosophical, or practical approaches and also can be oriented empirically or nonempirically (not that those two categories are always mutually exclusive). As ways of thinking, models can be stipulated or merely evident in the positions and arguments expressed by nurses.

SUGGESTED MODELS FOR KNOWLEDGE DEVELOPMENT

A variety of different foci are offered to stimulate knowledge development and provoke thought on the potential for nursing. In this chapter, philosophical concerns, such as identifying the goals and criteria for progress in nursing, and specific aims for inquiry, such as theory or concept development, are included as areas for furthering knowledge development in nursing. Nurses also are encouraged to consider the potential of human-centered forms of inquiry, such as the

---

BOX 13-1

SELECTED TYPES OF MODELS

Symbolic model	Conceptual model
Analog model	Heuristic model

study of experience and story, and to incorporate a focus on the contexts in which humans live and the critique of discourse and ideology. The topics addressed by no means represent an exhaustive list of possibilities nor are they presented in any order of priority. They are offered as potentially fruitful areas for consideration to stimulate knowledge development activity in the field.

Identifying Goals, Criteria, and Ideas of Progress

Inquiry to identify goals for the discipline of nursing as well as definitions of progress and criteria for determining progress could be beneficial in all knowledge development activities in nursing. The purpose of such activity would not be to apply a rational view to the development of nursing "science." Attempts to distinguish between science and other forms of knowledge can be more confusing than constructive. The adoption of principles of rational science might give the impression that the only concern is *science* because this idea of rational processes generally is not seen in regard to other types of knowledge.

In spite of the association of ideas of progress and criteria with a rational view of science, nursing still could benefit from some notions associated with that approach. Identification of goals for the discipline (not merely goals for practice and education), the desired direction for growth (progress) in knowledge development, and some consensus on what criteria can be used to determine if nursing is advancing and moving in an appropriate direction can help in the creation of a cohesive body of knowledge. The tremendous range of possibilities for nursing can lead to confusion and a disorderly approach to knowledge; resources can be scattered and misdirected when goals are not clear. The work that has been done in nursing, for example, in the areas of health promotion, behavior change, client education, and pain management, create a strong sense of progress and orderliness where advances in knowledge are evident and easier to apply in many cases. Nurses should never be stifled in efforts to be creative and innovative, to tackle new problems as they are encountered, or to try new solutions or paths. Nonetheless, the ability to see similarity, overlap, direction, meaning, and utility in the development of nursing knowledge in general could do a great deal to promote progress in the discipline as a whole.

Theory-Oriented Development

Theory development and testing has been an important focus of "science" and of nursing inquiry since the 1970s. The Logical Positivist movement initially stimulated this emphasis. One primary tenet of this view held that the development of theory was the proper goal of a science. In addition according to this view, the existence of theory was the defining characteristic in differentiating "science" from "non-science" in regard to knowledge.

Early in the movement to promote theory development in nursing, primary emphasis was placed on **grand theory** that would portray the nature and functions of nursing. Nurse theorists at the time seemed to strive for **formal** theory to the extent possible, attempting to show axiomatic relationships among components of the theory (Hardy, 1978). Martha Rogers' (1970) work on the theoretical basis of nursing practice presents a formula for the process of human development similar to the type of symbolic logic desired by the Logical Positivists. **Metatheory**, or discussion on the nature of theory, means of theory construction, and criteria for evaluation of theory also were significant topics for discussion while nurses learned how to develop theory for their own discipline.

The emphasis on theory in nursing has shifted radically over the years since that initial foray into theory development. Theories developed during this time have survived and continue to provide important perspectives on nursing for many clinical settings and educational programs. As time passed, however, the focus increasingly has been on the theory's usefulness as a guide for practice or as a means to generate explanations for various situations. One aspect of this shift is evident in discussions about theory "of" versus theory "for" nursing. Barrett (1991) describes this debate, showing the initial differentiation of "theory of" versus "theory for" in regard to the original source of the knowledge. According to Barrett, theory "of" was applied to theory originating or emanating from nursing, or theory that was new and original to the discipline. Theory "for" referred to theory that resulted from a synthesis of knowledge derived from other disciplines yet was applicable to nursing practice (p. 48). In this view, theory "of" nursing means theory created by nurses for their own purposes and use.

This debate can be reframed in a manner consistent with current needs and trends. In examining the structure of the phrase "theory of nursing," it is easy to think of theory that describes or explains how nursing works and the roles of nurses and their interactions with clients. This also might be referred to as theory "about" nursing. Theory for nursing is not limited to theory created in other disciplines. Instead it could refer generally to theory that is relevant to guide nursing practice, in other words, theory that is useful in nursing activities.

Theory can take a variety of forms useful in nursing (Box 13-2). Grand theories are described by Higgins and Moore (2000) as

> the global paradigms of nursing science. They are formal, highly abstract theoretical systems that frame our disciplinary knowledge within the principles of nursing, and their concepts and propositions transcend specific events and patient populations. (p. 180)

Grand theories are abstract and tend to provide broad explanations or characterizations of nursing. They do not provide the specific information essential to determine appropriate actions on the part of the nurse.

Sociologist Robert Merton (1957) described his idea of **middle-range theories** as being appropriate to guide research and specific enough to guide practice for nursing. The level of abstraction evident in grand theories makes it difficult if not impossible to subject them to the usual modes of "testing." They are not purported to be true or false but are more of a philosophical perspective on a situa-

BOX 13-2

LEVELS OF THEORY

Grand theory	Micro-range theory
Middle-range theory	Situation-specific theory

tion. In contrast to grand theories, middle-range theories are narrower in scope as well as less abstract. There is, therefore, more potential for applying them in real-world situations.

Middle-range theories currently have the most emphasis in nursing. The possibility of testing and the ease with which such theories can be applied in nursing practice account for this emphasis. Another category that includes theories even narrower in scope also has attracted nurses' attention for the same reasons. Higgins and Moore (2000) describe **micro-range theory** as "the most restrictive in terms of time and scope or application" (p. 181). According to these authors, micro-range theories are more "tentative" than the grand and middle-range theories and serve as a means to test working hypotheses so they can be developed into a more organized theoretical system. Im and Meleis (1999) propose a form of theory they refer to as "situation-specific" in regard to theories that have a narrow range of application yet lack the tentativeness of the micro-range theory. A **situation-specific theory** applies only in very limited circumstances due to the narrow scope of the theory.

This brief discussion of levels of theory points out that activity to develop theory in nursing is an important part of knowledge development activity and continues to be the focus of considerable discussion. Theory serves as an important mechanism for organizing knowledge. Theory enables the nurse to move from one situation to the next with knowledge of concepts and relationships that can be applied in multiple encounters. Without theory, each situation in which the nurse is engaged would seem unique or new, as if the nurse were seeing it for the first time. Organizing knowledge into some form regardless of the level of the theoretical product provides information that can be carried, applied, and evaluated from case to case. As a result, the nurse enters situations with some established ideas and ways of viewing the situation that help to provide initial understanding of the events that are taking place.

Fawcett's (1978) seminal article describing the close relationship between theory and research still has relevance in nursing knowledge development. Fawcett described this relationship using the metaphor of the double helix construction of DNA to show how closely intertwined these two components of knowledge development must be for effective outcomes. At the time of the publication of this article and into the early 1980s, there was an overwhelming emphasis on theory development as the primary need of the discipline. While knowledge development now can be seen as much broader than theory development alone, there still is much to be gained by pursuing theory-building activities. The usefulness of theory, discussed previously, reveals the advantages of continuing research to develop, refine, and expand the theories available to guide nursing activity. Theory development work also serves to organize nursing knowledge, making it possible to promote growth and progress in the discipline. By synthesizing knowledge into the forms of theory regardless of level, a cohesive body of knowledge can be seen that is relevant and applicable to nursing.

The phrases "theory testing" and "theory development" are likely to conjure images of experimental designs, randomized trials, or other similar forms of research. It is important to remember that, in addition to the levels of theory described previously, theory can exist in a variety of forms including descriptive. As the name implies, **descriptive theory** provides a description of what is happening in a situation and reveals the components that exist in a situation such as the elements of the experience encountered by significant others of persons living with AIDS (Cowles & Rodgers, 1991) or family members placing an older adult in a nursing home (Rodgers, 1997). Numerous similar instances of theory development can be found in the literature of nursing as well as in other fields. Such theories can be developed using qualitative methods particularly the method of Grounded Theory (Glaser & Strauss, 1967). Quint (1967) made the case for theories created in this manner, which are generated from empirical data, in the late 1960s to show alternatives to the more widely understood processes of hypothesis testing as a means to develop theory.

Theories can be more loosely organized collections of concepts or constructs, such as the case with descriptive theories. These theories reveal the substance of a situation yet without structured linkages showing the specific nature of relationships among components. Theories also can be developed inductively or deductively through a process of rational reconstruction of situations based on experience or observation or through systematic deduction of hypotheses and testing. Parts of theories can be explored further to clarify vague aspects or to identify the scope of contexts in which it is reasonable to apply the theory. Theories, as a result, may move progressively toward a more formal end of the continuum because relational statements are refined to the point that they take the form of propositions. In the process of theory development, it is important not to expect all theory to be moved to a formal level. The value of descriptive, substantive theory easily can be overlooked in such a scheme. Descriptive theory offers a great deal to nurses who need some idea of what might be taking place in a situation as well as the flexibility to view each encounter with enough openness to accommodate the tremendous diversity of humans and their experiences.

Concept Development

Concept development provides another means to expand the knowledge base of nursing and a worthwhile activity for nursing inquiry. Concept development has not received the attention it deserves as an important mechanism for knowledge development. This may be due partly to consideration given to the more familiar realm of theory development. The value of concept development also may not be appreciated due to an abundance of "concept analysis" reports based on unclear or untenable philosophical assumptions. As a result, the potentially vital contributions of concept development to enhancing the knowledge base and to application in nursing situations may not be apparent.

It is reasonable to argue that all inquiry in some sense is a form of concept development. Research to identify interventions for pain contributes to a better understanding of pain as a concept. An instrument developed to measure grief or autonomy or job satisfaction contributes to a greater understanding of those concepts. A broad conceptual process takes place when a researcher observes something, gives a word label to that phenomenon, and uses that word to communicate and share ideas with others. Nursing can advance through careful attention to the conceptual roots of knowledge and focused work to develop useful, applicable, and less ambiguous concepts (Rodgers, 2000).

Concept development occurs using both conceptual and empirical processes. As noted above, measurement and instrumentation are closely linked to concept development. Literature-based analyses can be used to determine the current status of a concept as well as to identify alternative ways of thinking about a situation. Westra and Rodgers' (1991) work on the concept of integration serves as an excellent example of the development of new concepts for use in nursing. Westra identified a number of limitations with the concept of adaptation, which had been used to reflect the processes that older adults experience when learning to live with chronic conditions. A literature-based analysis initially was used to determine the potential for the concept of integration to reflect more accurately the experiences of the members of the population. In conducting this inquiry, Westra combined her familiarity with the extant literature on this situation with her own observations followed by lengthy literature review to discover and eventually develop an alternative. By conceptualizing the situation as an example of integration rather than adaptation, Westra and Rodgers shift the focus from an individual who has to learn to deal with limitations or specific needs to one who creates a new sense of self. This example shows the potential power of concepts and language in addition to merely showing the utility of the method.

The importance of concept development in the expansion of nursing knowledge served as a focal point for the philosophy of Toulmin (1972). Toulmin saw the scientific enterprise consisting primarily of a process of expanding, enhancing, and clarifying the conceptual repertoire of the field. This view gives nurses additional reason to consider the potential for concept-related activities in developing the knowledge base of nursing.

Experience, Story, and Narrative

The development of nursing knowledge requires understanding each person's uniqueness and individual experiences. In the Empiricist era, "experience" applied exclusively to "sensory experience." Perhaps following the lead of Kant, the phenomenologists, and more recently the postmodernists, human **experience** is viewed in a broader, whole-person sense, in other words, as a totality of emotions, feelings, sensations, and life changes associated with some occurrence.

Decades of debate have taken place in nursing, as in many other disciplines, regarding the value of various methods to capture individual experiences. The use of qualitative means to capture individual experiences still generates some discussion in "scientific" circles. Some of this debate stems from traditional notions of "science" and a preoccupation with science over a more general concern for "knowledge."

The important consideration in this regard for nursing and in the context of this text concerns the philosophical basis for examining experience. Methods are available to study just about anything imaginable. The key to quality and meaningful inquiry, however, lies with understanding the philosophical underpinnings of the method, in other words, what does it "mean" to study something a particular way. It is also relevant to consider the way in which the research fits with or contributes to the development of the discipline's knowledge base.

Personal experience constitutes an important component of nursing consideration in working with individuals. Statistical projections of outcomes regarding medication effectiveness, symptom relief, and extension of life are valuable but do not provide a complete picture of the anticipated individual situation in regard to personal functioning, side effects, or impact on family and other personal relationships. Research has shown, however, that such factors are very important to people when making decisions about treatment or care. Research also has shown that individuals have their own decision-making styles and use data from various sources differently in sorting through options. Kelly-Powell's (1997) study of decision making regarding treatment by people with life-threatening conditions mirrored the decision-making style they used in other situations. Anecdotal, personal, statistical, physician-provided, and other sources of data are given different weight and consideration according to the individual's cognitive style. In many cases, personal knowledge of what happened with a neighbor or family member or coworker in a situation similar to their own is more important than empirical data provided by health care professionals. Instrumentation is not available to study many psychosocial experiences and it may not be appropriate in all instances. Along with some changes in philosophy and ideas about science, these observations have helped to create a context in which methods other than those of traditional science need to be pursued.

Narratives, story, and **discourse** are important tools in the quest to understand human experience. The terms narrative and story often are used in the same context in regard to research. Drawing on the narrative theory of Ricouer (1984), narrative inquiry actually comprises a distinct realm of research. Narrative inquiry in general involves the collection of detailed descriptions of an experience provided by an individual. These narratives can be examined for common themes or divided into separate "stories" then analyzed for the themes presented within each story. A philosophical assumption underlying the idea of **story** in inquiry consists of the idea that people understand and interpret their lives in the form of stories. According to this way of thinking, human beings construct their lives and make sense of them by forming stories from their experiences. In narrative inquiry, the investigator typically uses interview techniques to elicit detailed descriptions of an experience by a participant; the researcher or interviewer often allows the individual to talk quite freely with only minimal direction or guidance. Telling stories provides a depth of detail and insight that cannot be obtained through structured means (Frid, Öhlén, & Bergbom, 2000; Kennedy, Shannon, Chuahorm, & Kravetz, 2004; Sakalys, 2003).

Bartol (1989) provides a different perspective on the use of story in the context of gathering information from a person about his or her history. Rather than stories being merely a "product of the imagination" (p. 565) as is typically thought when someone is "telling stories," Bartol points out that story is a potentially "more viable medium of communicating the truth than any objective analysis of extracted data can be" (p. 565). Storytelling in an active sense (not merely within the context of an extended research interview) can provide a depth of understanding and insight into the individual "meaning" of a situation; this is in contrast to presenting emphasis on the "facts" of the situation. A story also provides a means of self-knowledge for the storyteller because "very often, in the process of telling a story we discover new connections and gain insight into ourselves" (Bartol, 1989, p. 565).

Other forms of inquiry beyond the usual administration of research instruments warrant consideration and additional development in nursing. While narrative and story-related approaches are getting some consideration in nursing, methodologies can be developed that focus on other forms of expression such as dance and music. Art also holds significant promise as an expressive medium and has been used in studies with children and studies concerning violence and abuse among other topics of inquiry. Literature and literary analysis also warrant exploration as ways to capture aspects of human existence that do not lend themselves to reductionistic approaches but instead require methods that capture the broad range of an experience with more specific information and emotional components intact. Dance has been used to portray the experiences of persons living with terminal illness and warrants attention to determine its potential as a possible means of nursing inquiry, learning, and experiencing. The future of nursing knowledge development will be enhanced considerably not only by the expanded application of currently accepted methods but also by the development of new approaches to understand and interpret human experience.

Context and Criticism

Although not the last of possible directions that seem fruitful for nursing knowledge development, the final one that will be addressed here concerns attention to context and social criticism. As evident in previous chapters addressing postmodernism and feminism, some philosophers emphasize that social context has tremendous effect on each individual; social context factors include economics, class, ethnicity, gender, family structure, and education.. These factors also affect the value system and perspectives that each investigator brings to the research situation. Even the most rigorous empirical study needs to be evaluated in regard to contextual elements that might have affected the findings or might have an influence on applicability in diverse settings.

Power is a significant component of nursing and health care situations. Even though nurses may see themselves as acting in the best interest of the client or being in the position of client advocate, clients may still see the nurse as a figure with power and authority. The notion of advocacy carries a sense of a power differential, placing the nurse in a privileged position in regard to the remainder of the health care system. The roles of power and authority can be explored in a variety of ways including analysis of communication and publications (discourse) as ways to uncover the aspects of this differential that may not be obvious to those involved.

Nurses need to consider the clients' expectations, needs, and perspective as well as the nurse's perspective or any theoretical basis from which the nurse operates. Awareness of literature, educational materials, and advertisements that can affect the person's expectations and preconceptions can be quite revealing as the nurse attempts to establish relationships with clients and their significant others; knowing the client's preferences can help the nurse to select and present effective and useful information for treatment and for decision making. Discourse analysis can provide insight into the obvious messages present in communication and the hidden meanings that influence the perceptions of recipients of care; this analysis also can shed light on the nurse's own behaviors and presuppositions.

CONCLUSION

A wide variety of methods and models are available for nursing knowledge development. Some have been described in this chapter particularly to shed light on some significant areas for further research. One objective in nursing knowledge development can be the desire to progress in a more compact manner, promoting organized and internally coherent knowledge development efforts that are complementary and mutually beneficial to all involved including researchers and recipients of care. Awareness of changes in methodology, development of new methodologies, and expansion and testing currently available means for inquiry can stimulate further development in nursing and perhaps speed the acquisition of comprehensive knowledge systems. The approaches discussed in this chapter—theory development, concept development, attention to experience and narrative, and consideration of diverse contexts—have potentially important roles in focusing knowledge development efforts. Nurses also should work to develop new methodologies and new ways of knowing along with exploring the criteria and means for creating defensible arguments for knowledge claims. Working from the foundation provided by a combination of approaches designed to obtain unique knowledge goals can give nurses new insights into ways to provide the knowledge that is needed in the discipline and that can effectively address nursing problems.

 # FOR DISCUSSION

1. Identify a goal appropriate to direct knowledge development efforts in nursing.
2. Describe criteria that would be appropriate to determine progress in achieving the goals of nursing.
3. Discuss the differences among metatheory, grand theory, middle-range theory, and micro-range theory in application to nursing.
4. Discuss a focus in nursing in which concept development would be appropriate to advance the knowledge base of nursing.
5. Discuss ways in which techniques of critique or social criticism can be useful to expand the knowledge base of nursing.

REFERENCES

Barrett, E. M. (1991). Theory: Of or for nursing? *Nursing Science Quarterly, 4*(2), 48–49.

Bartol, B. M. (1989). Story in nursing practice. *Nursing and Health Care, 10,* 564–565.

Cody, W. K. (1999). Middle-range theories: Do they foster the development of nursing science? *Nursing Science Quarterly, 12,* 9–14.

Cowles, K. V., & Rodgers, B. L. (1991). When a loved one has AIDS: Care for the significant other. *Journal of Psychosocial Nursing and Mental Health Services, 29*(4), 6–12.

Fawcett, J. (1978). The relationship between theory and research: A double helix. *Advances in Nursing Science, 1*(1), 49–62.

Frid, I., Öhlén, J., & Bergbom, I. (2000). On the use of narratives in nursing research. *Journal of Advanced Nursing, 32,* 695–703.

Glaser, B. G., & Strauss, A. L. (1967). *The discovery of grounded theory: Strategies for qualitative research.* Chicago: Aldine.

Hardy, M. E. (1978). Perspectives on nursing theory. *Advances in Nursing Science, 1*(1), 27–48.

Higgins, P. A., & Moore, S. M. (2000). Levels of theoretical thinking in nursing. *Nursing Outlook, 48,* 179–183.

Im, E-O., & Meleis, A. I. (1999). Situation-specific theories: Philosophical roots, properties, and approach. *Advances in Nursing Science, 22,* 11–24.

Kelly-Powell, M. (1997). Personalizing choices: Patients' experiences with making treatment decisions. *Research in Nursing and Health, 20,* 219–227.

Kennedy, H. P., Shannon, M. T., Chuahorm, U., & Kravetz, M. K. (2004). The landscape of caring for women: A narrative study of midwifery practice. *Journal of Midwifery and Women's Health, 49*(1), 14–23.

Merton, R. K. (1957). *Social theory and social structure.* NY: Free Press.

Quint, J. C. (1967). The case for theories generated from empirical data. *Nursing Research, 16,* 109–114.

Ricoeur, P. (1984). *Time and narrative* (K. McLaughlin and D. Pellauer, Trans.). Chicago: University of Chicago Press.

Rodgers, B. L. (1997). Family members' experiences with the nursing home placement of an older adult. *Applied Nursing Research, 10*(2), 57–63.

Rodgers, B. L. (2000). Philosophical foundations of concept development. In B. L. Rodgers & K. A. Knafl (Eds.), *Concept development in nursing: Foundations, techniques, and applications* (2nd Ed.) (pp. 7–38). Philadelphia: W. B. Saunders.

Rogers, M. (1970). *An introduction to the theoretical basis of nursing.* Philadelphia: F. A. Davis.

Sakalys, J. A. (2003). Restoring the patient's voice: The therapeutics of illness narratives. *Journal of Holistic Nursing, 21,* 228–241.

Toulmin, S. (1972). *Human understanding.* Princeton, NJ: Princeton University Press.

Westra, B. L., & Rodgers, B. L. (1991). The concept of integration: A foundation for evaluating outcomes of nursing care. *Journal of Professional Nursing, 5,* 277–282.

CHAPTER 14

The Future of Nursing Knowledge

KEY IDEAS

central concepts of nursing   international nursing
domains of nursing   substantive structure of a discipline
ecological focus of nursing   syntax of a discipline
environment

Discussing the future of nursing knowledge development involves a considerable amount of irony. People who proclaim to be able to predict what will happen in the future occasionally appear at nursing events or present their writings in the nursing literature as a way to share their visions. People who refer to themselves as "futurists" are popular speakers both for nursing and for the general public. It likely is part of human nature to want to know what to expect and consequently to be prepared for it when it happens. Those people whose predictions are a bit more accurate than the ideas of others are perhaps more adept at spotting trends. Predictions are heavily dependent on context, however, and the rapidly changing nature of the situations in which people live and grow means that even seemingly steadfast trends can be fleeting.

The irony in looking at the future stems not only from this difficult complex of context and predictability but also from the fact that those who share their visions of the future are also helping to create it. By saying that the future holds a particular focus for nursing, there is some possibility that such a statement will steer work in that particular direction. The future of nursing knowledge, therefore, is something to be created not something to be predicted.

Promoting continuing progress and growth in nursing requires more than just a vision of the desired future; it requires the awareness and skills needed to achieve that vision. An understanding of philosophy along with dialectic reasoning skills can be very beneficial in moving forward with nursing knowledge development. Philosophy underlies everything; in knowledge development, it provides the view and a focus for understanding the world and the human beings in it. It provides perspectives on how to understand or "know" anything about the world, and it provides means to evaluate the knowledge that is created. It also provides the basis for the values that drive decision making in regard to knowledge development such as in the determination of priorities and the selection of modes of inquiry to be pursued. All of these, in turn, need to be evaluated for their appropriateness and relevance to the development of the knowledge base for nursing. Over time, development of skills to conduct this sort of critical analysis will serve nurses better than learning the names and specific contributions of various philosophers.

Philosophy also shapes, as well as describes, human endeavors. In this text, an intellectual history approach was pursued to show some of the major traditions in Western philosophy. Although nurses have not necessarily drawn ideas directly from the writings of early philosophers, their works certainly have shaped the culture and the ideas of knowledge that have influenced nursing ideology. In the 1970s and into the early 1990s, the primary emphasis in nursing was on the development of "science" as a highly specialized and particularly esteemed form of knowledge. Nursing's journey into knowledge development owes a great deal to that movement to develop "science." While this focus may seem to have sidetracked efforts to build a knowledge base in the discipline, it does constitute an important period in the development of the discipline. The desire of nurses to have the discipline viewed as a "science" was coupled with a growth in graduate and particularly doctoral level education in nursing, the procurement of federal funds to support nursing education and research, and the advent of several of the prominent research publications in nursing. Perhaps most important in regard to the focus here, it marks the beginning of nursing's exploration of philosophy, science, and theory development. The quest to develop an epistemic focus in nursing, or a basis for understanding how nurses know, what counts as knowledge in nursing, and how nurses can are best able to create the knowledge needed has an obvious tie to this period of the 1960s and 1970s.

This phase in the history of nursing subsequently led to some critical analysis of the dominant ideology of the time. Some scholars in other disciplines began to question the appropriateness and the utility of views of knowledge as they were presented in the literature, and nurses' connections with other disciplines enabled some of the newer ideas to filter into the nursing literature. Nurse scholars undoubtedly found it important to keep up with changing views in philosophy on their own. Nurses began writing about paradigms (Conway, 1985; Hardy, 1978; Kim, 1989) in addition to theories as the work of Kuhn gained popularity; this discussion ultimately included consideration of the nature of nursing as a discipline, ways of knowing, postmodern ideology, and contextual considerations relevant to nursing knowledge.

Nursing has evolved to include more graduate education programs, more nurses with doctoral level education in nursing, a variety of doctoral degrees, more opportunities and resources to support research, and a greater role in the creation of health care related knowledge. In the midst of such growth, it may be tempting to avoid spending time contemplating the nature of the work and the knowledge base of nursing and to simply get on with doing the work of nursing. However, that approach cannot serve the needs of nursing to ensure effective problem solving and progress and the coherent growth of the discipline. In addition, ongoing critique and analysis are essential to ensure that nursing continues to be relevant in changing social, political, economic, and care delivery contexts.

Nurses need not only to evaluate and critically analyze available options for knowledge development; scholars and leaders in the field need to be involved in creating new approaches and modes of inquiry and revising visions of nursing to promote continuing development. No single existing philosophy is likely to be wholly satisfactory to meet the needs of nurse scholars and the discipline. Nurses will need to modify, adapt, or expand philosophical ideology and explore the applicability of various approaches to knowledge development. Because philosophers in general do not write for a particular discipline, nurses will need to evaluate approaches and share their ideas and interpretations to promote philosophically sound growth in the field. While nurses are actively doing the research necessary to expand the knowledge base, work on the philosophical side must continue to guide that work.

Some areas are apparent where work might be particularly valuable in nursing. As the nature of health care continues to change, nurses can benefit from reexamining their roles and how they approach their work and the development of knowledge in regard to the conceptualization of the discipline. Reconsideration of the **domains of nursing**, the variety of philosophical perspectives available to guide knowledge development, and the possibility of new methods to develop knowledge can significantly promote growth in the discipline (Box 14-1).

DOMAINS OF NURSING

Since the beginning of efforts to delineate an identifiable body of nursing knowledge, nurses have focused on specific content as comprising the discipline of nursing. The report by Yura and Torres (1975) regarding a survey of baccalaureate programs conducted by the National League for Nursing demonstrated that the central concepts in nursing were man (sic), nursing, health, and society. This list was revised by Fawcett (1978) who used the terms "person" instead of "man," and "environment" instead of "society," to present a broader view of these components in nursing. Other authors introduced variations on these concepts (Stevens, 1979),

> ### BOX 14-1
>
> ## FUTURE VISION OF NURSING
>
> - Revision of criteria for the domains of nursing
> - Expansion of environment domain and ecological focus
> - Incorporation of changing philosophies
> - Refinement of methodologies
> - Creation of new methods to reflect changing philosophies

particularly the nurse theorists who provided detailed depictions of human development and health and wellness. Kim (1987) also recognized this pattern of conceptual agreement in nursing. Stimulated by the move toward taxonomy development, she constructed a typology of four domains intended to provide some structure for the development of nursing knowledge. These domains addressed the client, the interaction of the client and nurse, nursing practice, and the environment.

These attempts to identify the core of nursing were consistent with earlier efforts to resolve what Donaldson and Crowley (1978) referred to in another classic article as "the problem that plagues all of us: identification of the essence of nursing research and of the common elements and threads that give coherence to an identifiable body of knowledge" (p. 113). Donaldson and Crowley stated further that the emphasis of nursing tended to involve a "tacit rather than explicit knowledge of the broad conceptualizations unique to nursing" (p. 113). In other words, there might be a core of content associated with nursing yet that knowledge base needed to be developed and articulated more directly and clearly.

Donaldson and Crowley provided a schema of how disciplines are constructed; they draw on the prevailing educational philosophy of Shermis (1962) and Schwab (1964). This approach distinguishes each discipline according to unique **syntax** (or ways of knowing) and **substantive structure** (content). It is evident they did not intend to draw distinct boundaries around disciplines. Donaldson and Crowley devoted considerable discussion to the interrelatedness of the disciplines and how the development of one discipline may have some relationship to the development of others. The hierarchical view of knowledge supported by Comte (1953) and the Logical Positivists contributed somewhat to this idea. Nonetheless, Donaldson and Crowley cautioned nurses not to rely on other disciplines to develop the knowledge needed to guide their actions. Instead they argued that researchers prepared to conduct inquiry consistent with the needs and perspective of nursing should be engaged in building the knowledge base appropriate to the discipline.

Since this foundation, the domains have persisted as reflecting the relevant concerns of nursing. On cursory examination, there is considerable reason to continue to adhere to these ideas about the substantive focus of nursing. Despite the limited resources available within the care delivery or practice domain, nurses work with people, establish what are presumably therapeutic relationships, and incorporate information about the person's environment in assessing needs and possibilities.

Moving beyond this past and expanding the knowledge base and the potential for nursing seem to warrant reconsideration of these domains at present. Nursing particularly needs to expand the concepts of client and environment. In some instances, nurses may find that the environment is a more appropriate focus of intervention than a person or aggregate of people.

Nurses and the Environment

Nurses generally are aware of the impact of the **environment** on the well-being of individuals. Older adults and others with physical needs might be taught ways to alter the environment to make some tasks easier as well as to facilitate mobility and increase safety. Similarly the link between air pollution and respiratory diseases such as emphysema and asthma is common knowledge in nursing; the negative effects of second-hand smoke on the health of adults and children are also well known. People with respiratory conditions might be taught how to manage their activity according to climate and pollution conditions, to use air filters or air conditioners to clean the air entering their work or living spaces, and how to avoid noxious stimuli that might exacerbate their individual conditions.

While these interventions are completely appropriate and part of the usual care provided by nurses, they affect only the individual living in the particular situation. These examples show how care is focused on helping the person adapt to an unhealthy environment as exemplified through the use of air filters and avoidance. While such suggestions are beneficial to the individual, they do nothing to address the actual problem, which is a problem of the broader community and the environment.

Environmental problems account for a substantial number of illnesses, lost wages, health care costs, early death, and disability. Environmental problems cannot be left to the arena of public health, politics, or environmental action groups to solve. Nurses have an incredible opportunity to take an active role in improving society's health and well-being, decreasing incidence of disease or improving quality of life, and providing a more healthy ecological system through an expanded focus on the client. Comprehensive and improved health is the target of nursing care and includes the environment as a significant component of nursing practice (Box 14-2).

Nurses are in an ideal position to assess common environmental hazards and provide educational programs to promote healthier environments. Nurses can identify problems, educate about hazards, provide information and testimony during political processes, help to identify alternatives, and interpret research for oth-

---

BOX 14-2

EXAMPLES OF NURSING FOCI WITHIN THE ENVIRONMENT DOMAIN

- Environment as a focus of nursing intervention
- Maintenance of healthy ecosystems
- Food safety
- Social problems
- Economic barriers

---

ers. The importance of balanced and healthy ecosystems, in which the focus is on keeping the system of living things in balance for any part to thrive, is becoming increasingly obvious as critical to the achievement of health and well-being. Food safety has recently received considerable attention as an important part of this effort. In fact, environmental quality has been identified in the Healthy People initiative as one of the leading health indicators. These indicators reflect what are considered to be the most important health concerns in the United States; they include a variety of behavioral, social, and economic factors linked to human health (U.S. Department of Health and Human Services, 2000).

Nurses can take an active role in improving physical, social, and economic environments and in increasing knowledge about the relationships between these elements and human health. A central focus of nursing continues to be the ability to see individuals in a broader light, in other words, how people live with the conditions and resources available to them. Nurses, as a result, should be an important component in the effort to help people and communities adopt healthy habits and lifestyles and to help match individual goals to larger community and environmental health.

The environment also includes the larger ecological system not just issues affecting air, water, and pesticide use. Nurses in recent history have taken pride in their holistic focus in dealing with individuals. It is reasonable and timely for nurses to expand this view to a broader ecological focus. As awareness grows of the interconnectedness of people with other elements on the planet, this holistic perspective needs to be expanded to appreciate fully the position of people relative to the entire environment around them as the key to well-being. Due to the synergistic nature of all life, this idea of environment needs to include attention to living things besides people. Nurses have an outstanding opportunity to expand their perspective and scope to include the environment as a direct recipient of nursing intervention and to promote an ecological focus in health care. Acting on such a level can have far greater positive impact on health and well-being than acting only on the individual level.

The early 21st century is an optimal time for nurses to expand their potential to this broader level. Medical treatment and reimbursement are constantly changing and chronic illness and lifestyle related problems are increasing; an emphasis on general well-being and prevention could not be more timely. As nurses seek expanded roles and opportunities outside the acute care setting, a more holistic, ecological model emphasizing a broader concept of client and an expanded environment domain could serve nursing and the public well into the future.

EXPANDING PHILOSOPHICAL AWARENESS

The future of nursing also can be expected to include an increased focus on international health and nursing. Exchanges between countries are becoming common for both students and teachers, and Western expertise is called upon frequently as a model for care in other parts of the world. Journals have become increasingly international in focus and published articles reflect growing attention to health issues in a multitude of countries.

It is difficult to dismiss the need to expand the vision of nursing to include broader consideration of the large systems in which humans live and interact. Just as this expanded perspective applies to the environment, it applies across the planet to diverse cultures and settings. Opportunities for knowledge development in the future need to be structured so as to benefit from this broader perspective. One danger in the internationalization of knowledge is that dominant cultures and views can be transported to other contexts where those views are not appropriate. For example, the dominant role of Western nursing and health care in shaping care in other systems could lead to the imparting of Western values and ways of practice in other parts of the world. As a result, the strengths and richness of these other contexts might be undermined. Knowledge development in nursing needs to proceed from a basis of creating an effective exchange with nurses learning from the principles and philosophies of health that underlie care in different contexts. The homogenization of knowledge and practice models should be avoided. At present, it is not uncommon to see alternative modes of care transplanted without regard to philosophy; acupuncture or Chinese herbs might be interpreted within a Western allopathic model of treatment, becoming only another possible intervention to consider. Interventions of this nature, however, are derived from a distinct philosophy of both health and human existence. Failure to recognize this connection may undermine the outcomes of treatment and deprive recipients of the maximum benefit of care. Such an approach also reinforces that the current thinking about health care is appropriate and perpetuates existing models of health and health care delivery rather than fully integrating new approaches.

Health care is evolving on a constant basis. New technologies are incorporated rapidly in the interest of improving care while also decreasing monetary and ideally human costs. At the same time, nursing and health care operate within a social context that also changes continually, presenting new expectations and demands for care. Information diffusion has accelerated in recent years, enabling people to

> ### BOX 14-3
>
> ## EXAMPLES OF METHODOLOGICAL ADVANCES
>
> - Methods based on philosophies other than traditional "Western"
> - Refinement of current methods
> - New methods developed appropriate to revised and expanded domains
> - Nonempirical modes of inquiry
> - Development of criteria to evaluate quality of diverse modes of inquiry

be informed about possibilities and alternatives on a much greater level than ever before. This context overall calls for nursing knowledge development that is current, relevant, shows awareness of alternatives, and is based on a variety of philosophical positions. Eastern and Indian philosophies underlie a number of currently popular trends in health care particularly in regard to self-treatment and more recently the application of naturopathic remedies. Nursing's holistic focus could be a good fit with some of the ideas and principles of these philosophies. Nursing knowledge development needs to expand beyond the realm of Western philosophy to consider what can be gained from a broader perspective and to evaluate alternate philosophies for their potential epistemic contributions.

 ## METHODOLOGICAL ADVANCES

As philosophy about living and knowing changes, so must methodological work to remain consistent with new ideas and to take advantage of the new awareness created by changes in philosophy. Nursing knowledge development has been transformed since the 1980s to include a variety of qualitative methods; altered interpretations of "science" and traditional forms of research; and the incorporation of text, narrative, and discourse as ways of developing knowledge. There is still considerable room for growth and expansion in regard to methods of inquiry (Box 14-3).

Existing methods need to be refined continually to provide approaches that are consistent with evolving philosophy and that provide the best means to achieve the goals of the discipline. As nursing expands its conceptualizations of environment and client, new approaches will be needed to capture emerging phenomena and the new concepts created to characterize these phenomena. A particular need will exist for ways to capture the complexity of existence and the interactions of multiple systems as they affect health and well-being and to avoid the reductionism seemingly inherent in any attempt at inquiry. A focus on empirical realms of knowing limits knowledge development to elements that are sensory in nature or the historical attempt to transform nonempirical entities into something that can be captured using empirical means.

Aristotle confronted this same problem when dealing with the idea of the Platonic forms, which are clearly nonempirical elements that seemed to lie beyond human grasp. Aristotle attempted to show how such nonempirical elements could be found in everyday objects and how the nature of the nonempirical elements could be demonstrated by combining observations with existing truths. His approach was unique for its combination of logical thought with sensory data. While his method certainly does not provide the ultimate answer for nursing's attempts to construct new methods for inquiry, it does reveal the potential of considering alternative ways of learning about people and the world in which they live.

Nurse researchers can learn a great deal by further examination of nonempirical methods of inquiry and expression; the time would seem ripe to explore the potential for these alternative approaches to knowledge. Music, dance, and art have been demonstrated to be valuable means of expression and are used as therapies in some situations. Movement, dance, and voice therapy are established interventions, complete with professional associations that provide new avenues to understanding and expressing the self. If these techniques can be used for self-understanding, then it is reasonable to consider exploring such approaches as ways of gaining knowledge that will be relevant to nursing.

The application of such methods, however, is likely to create new challenges in regard to criteria that can support results of such inquiry. Tangible evidence often is given the greatest weight in regard to substantiation of knowledge claims. Yet some elements of existence of greatest concern to nurses are inherently intangible. Means to capture these phenomena, provide supporting evidence, and construct defensible arguments need to be explored to take full advantage of the many potential ways of knowing and interacting with the world.

 ## CONCLUSION

Some of the philosophies presented in this text provide useful insight into how defensible arguments might be constructed in the future such as by focusing on problem solving (Laudan, 1977), enlightenment (Gadamer, 1975), power differentials (Foucault, 1972), and story and action (Ricoeur, 1981). Understanding these and other philosophies and being aware of new ideas that emerge in philosophy give nurses the skills needed for continuing successful knowledge development in the future. Knowledge development in nursing currently confronts numerous opportunities for expanding the way of looking at the world and the role of nurses in human existence. With solid skills of reasoning and critical analysis and with an open mind to possibilities as yet unknown, nursing can proceed toward developing knowledge that meets the needs of the discipline, that places knowledge at the forefront of human inquiry, and that has the potential to make significant contributions to the creation of positive environments and the promotion of human health.

◈ FOR DISCUSSION

1. Discuss the ideas of person, nursing, health, and environment and how these domains might evolve for nursing knowledge development in a future context.

2. Develop and articulate a vision for the future development of nursing knowledge. Include identification of priorities for both substance and methods for developing knowledge.

3. Describe how the ontologic view—the view of the nature of reality—espoused in nursing influences the continuing development of knowledge.

4. Discuss the potential for an expanded focus of nursing beyond the individual as a recipient of nursing care.

5. Discuss implications and issues associated with international development of nursing knowledge.

REFERENCES

Comte, A. (1953). *A general view of positivism.* (J. H. Bridges, Trans.). Stanford, CA: Academic Reprints.

Conway, M. E. (1985). Toward greater specificity in defining nursing's metaparadigm. *Advances in Nursing Science, 7*(4), 73–81.

Donaldson, S. K., & Crowley, D. M. (1978). The discipline of nursing. *Nursing Outlook, 26,* 113–120.

Fawcett, J. (1978). The what of theory development. In *Theory development: What, why, and how* (pp. 17–33). New York: National League for Nursing. (NLN Pub. No. 15-1708)

Foucault, M. (1972). *The archaeology of knowledge* (A. M. S. Smith, Trans.). New York: Pantheon Books.

Gadamer, H. (1975). *Truth and method* (G. Borden & J. Cumming, Trans.). New York: Seabury Press.

Hardy, M. E. (1978). Perspectives on nursing theory. *Advances in Nursing Science, 1*(1), 27–48.

Kim, H. S. (1987). Structuring the nursing knowledge system: A typology of four domains. *Scholarly Inquiry for Nursing Practice, 1*(2), 99–110.

Kim, H. S. (1989). Theoretical thinking in nursing: Problems and prospects. *Recent Advances in Nursing, 24,* 106–122.

Laudan, L. (1977). *Progress and its problems: Toward a theory of scientific growth.* Berkeley, CA: University of California Press.

Ricoeur, P. (1981). *Hermeneutics and human sciences: Essays on language, action and interpretation* (J. B. Thompson, Ed. and Trans.). New York: Cambridge University Press.

Schwab, J. (1964). Structure of the disciplines: Meaning and significances. In G. W. Ford & L. Pugno (Eds.), *The structure of knowledge and the curriculum.* Chicago: Rand McNally.

Shermis, S. (1962). On becoming an intellectual discipline. *Phi Delta Kappan, 44,* 84–86.

Stevens, B. (1979). *Nursing theory.* Boston: Little, Brown.

U.S. Department of Health and Human Services. (2000). *Healthy people 2010* (2nd ed.), 2 vols. Washington, DC: U.S. Government Printing Office.

Yura, H., & Torres, G. (1975). Today's conceptual framework within baccalaureate nursing programs. In *Faculty, curriculum development. Part 3: Conceptual framework: Its meaning and function* (pp. 17–25). New York: National League for Nursing (NLN Pub. No. 15-1558).

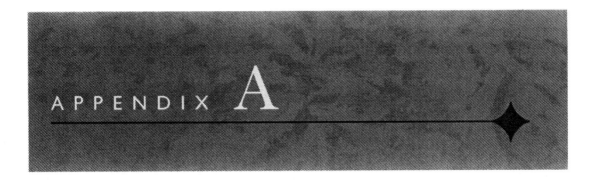

APPENDIX A

Philosophy Timeline

This philosophy timeline provides a broad frame of reference for the philosophies discussed in this text. The events listed were selected for their significance and because they are likely to be somewhat familiar to readers. This list is by no means reflective of the relative importance of any of these events or any events that are not listed. As is the case with knowledge, literature, art, and other human creations, philosophy both influences and is influenced by the context of the thinkers. Thus, the selected events and philosophies included here are intended to provide a reflection of major scientific, social, and cultural trends at the time. For further reading on history and philosophy, see the Internet Links provided in the Appendix.

APPENDIX

TIME	SIGNIFICANT PHILOSOPHY	SELECTED EVENTS
6th Century BCE	Thales, Anaximander, Anaximenes Pythagoras 581–497 BCE Confucius 557–479 BCE Heraclitus 540–460 BCE	Period of Ancient Greece Siddhartha (Gautama Buddha) born c. 563 BCE
5th Century BCE	Socrates 469–399 BCE Hippocrates c. 450–370 BCE	Persian Wars 500–451 BCE Peloponnesian War 450–401 BCE Parthenon completed 438 BCE Sophocles play, Oedipus, 429 BCE
4th Century BCE	Plato 428–347 BCE Aristotle 384–322 BCE Epicurus 340–271 BCE	Plato's Academy 380 BCE Aristotle's Lyceum 336 BCE
3rd–1st Cent. BCE	Stoicism Skepticism	Hellenistic Period (Golden Age of Greece) 360–340 BCE Roman Empire c. 146–380 BCE Greece conquered by Romans End of Chinese Classical Philosophy
1st–5th Cent. CE	Neo-Platonism Augustine 354–430 CE	Fall of Roman Empire c. 193–400 CE Rise of Christianity
6th–12th Cent. CE		Dark Ages 566–1100 Middle Ages 1000–1300 First crusade 1095 First universities founded: Bologna, 1113; Paris, 1150; Oxford, 1167 Genghis Khan 1162–1227
13th–15th Cent. CE	William of Ockham 1285–1349 Erasmus 1465–1536	Magna Carta 1215 Renaissance 1304–1576 Black Death, Europe 1347–1351 Byzantine Era ends; Constantinople falls 1453 Columbus crosses Atlantic 1492 DaVinci 1451–1519 Michelangelo 1475–1564 Luther (1483–1536) and German Reformation

APPENDIX

TIME	SIGNIFICANT PHILOSOPHY	SELECTED EVENTS

16th–18th Cent. CE	**Empiricism**
	Francis Bacon 1561–1626
	Locke 1632–1704
	Hume 1711–1776
	Berkeley 1685–1753
	
	Rationalism
	Descartes 1596–1650
	Spinoza 1632–1677
	
	Kantian Idealism
	Kant 1724–1804
	
	Idealism
	Schleiermacher 1768–1834
	Hegel 1779–1831
	Schopenhauer 1788–1860
		Queen Elizabeth I crowned 1558
		Copernicus 1473–1543
		First microscope 1590
		First telescope 1600
		Kepler 1571–1630, discovered elliptical
		   orbit of planets
		Philosophy written in native languages, not just
		   in Latin
		Harvey's study of circulation of blood 1628
		Galileo 1564–1642; inquisition 1633
		Newton 1642–1727
		Watt 1738–1819, invents steam engine
		Mary Wollstonecraft 1759–1797
		US Independence 1776

19th Century CE	**Positivism** Comte 1798–1857	Florence Nightingale 1820–1910 Seneca Falls Convention 1848 Crimean War 1854–1856 Freud 1856–1939 US Civil War 1862–1865

20th Century CE	**Philosophy of Science**
	
	Logical Positivism
	Schlick 1882–1936
	Mach 1838–1916
	Carnap 1891–1970
	Wittgenstein 1889–1951
	
	Historicism
	Kuhn 1922–1996
	Laudan 1941–
	Toulmin 1922–
	
	Phenomenology
	Husserl 1859–1938
	Merleau-Ponty 1908–1961
		Margaret Mead 1901–1978
		Bohr's theory of hydrogen atom 1913
		WW I 1914–1918
		Einstein's Relativity Theory 1915
		Women's suffrage movement 1916
		Mussolini in Italy 1922
		Equal rights amendment for women
		   first proposed 1923
		Lindbergh solo flight to Paris 1927
		Economic depression 1929
		Hitler takes power 1933
		Amelia Earhart lost during attempted
		   around the world flight 1937
		War of the Worlds radio broadcast 1938
		WW II 1939–1945
		FCC standard for Black and White
		   TV created 1941

APPENDIX

TIME	SIGNIFICANT PHILOSOPHY	SELECTED EVENTS
	Existentialism Heidegger 1889–1976 Sartre 1906–1980	Iron Curtain named 1946 Bell Laboratories creates the transistor 1947 Sputnik I and II satellites launched 1957
	Structuralism Levi-Strauss 1908-	NASA established 1958 Shepard's first US space flight 1961 Berlin wall 1961
	Critical Theory/ **Critical Social Theory** Marcuse 1898–1979 Adorno 1903–1969 Habermas 1929-	Cuban missile crisis 1962 Thalidomide linked to birth defects 1962 US enters Vietnam 1962 DDT banned in US 1969 First computer microprocessor 1971 Watergate break-in 1972
	Hermeneutics Gadamer 1900–2002	Billie Jean King defeats Bobby Riggs in tennis 1973 Microsoft founded 1975
	Poststructuralism and **Postmodernism** De Saussure 1857–1971 Foucault 1926–1984 Derrida 1930- Lyotard 1927–1998	National Academy of Sciences links spray can gases to changes in ozone 1976 Fall of the Berlin wall 1989–1990 Breakup of the Soviet Union c. 1991
	Feminism Elizabeth Cady Stanton 1815–1902 Simone de Beauvoir 1908–1986 Carol Gilligan 1936– Sandra Harding 1935–	

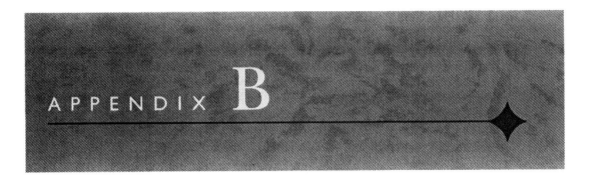

Biographical Statements
for Major Philosophers

Below are brief biographical statements for some of the philosophers featured in this text. The philosophers are fascinating not only for their work but also for their interesting and varied lives. A bibliography of selected reference sources is provided at the end for further reading.

ARISTOTLE 384–322 BCE

Born in Stagira on the Chalcidic peninsula in northern Greece, Aristotle had a father, Nichomachus, who was a physician and the doctor for Macedonian King Amyntas. Aristotle was 10 years of age when his father died; the boy was raised by a guardian, possibly an uncle. Aristotle acquired an interest in medicine and biology at an early age. He studied at Plato's Academy for 20 years, starting when he was 17 (367 BCE) and continuing until Plato's death. It is reported widely that Philip of Macedon invited Aristotle to tutor his son, Alexander (the Great), but there is debate about whether this actually occurred from 343 to 336 BCE. Aristotle went to Assos, Greece, where he worked with a group of philosophers collecting observations of zoological and biological natures. Aristotle founded his own philosophy school, the Lyceum, in 335. Charged with impiety in 323 and possibly fearing the same fate as Socrates, Aristotle fled to Chalcis and died there 1 year later.

FRANCIS BACON 1561–1626 CE

Born in London, England, into a prominent family with connections to royalty, Bacon was left impoverished after his father died in 1579. Bacon studied law, became a lawyer in 1582, entered the House of Commons in 1584, and was active in the prosecution of his long-time friend, the Earl of Essex, who was subsequently convicted as a traitor and executed. Bacon served as attorney general under James I and was knighted. Suffering economic problems most of his life, Bacon was charged with bribery, confessed, was convicted and imprisoned at the Tower of London for a short time then banished from Parliament and the court. He was subsequently pardoned and died in London in great debt.

RENE DESCARTES 1596–1650 CE

Born at Le Haye in Touraine, France, Descartes had a father who was a lawyer and magistrate. Descartes attended the Jesuit school La Flèche, where he became disenchanted with the traditional scholastic teachings of the classics and Aristotelian philosophy. Descartes received a degree in canon and civil law from the University of Poitiers. He joined the Bavarian Army in Holland in 1618 and traveled around Europe. He was invited by Queen Christina of Sweden to instruct her in philosophy in 1649. He died in 1650 presumably due partly to Sweden's cold climate and the Queen's demanding schedule.

MICHEL FOUCAULT 1926–1984 CE

Born in Poitiers, France, to a prominent local surgeon, Foucault generally was regarded as tormented but brilliant. He held a number of positions at universities in France. In 1969, he became Professor of the History of Systems of Thought at the prestigious Collège de France, where he remained until his death. Foucault was politically active and an outspoken advocate for members of marginalized groups. He was a frequent visiting professor or lecturer at universities in the United States and elsewhere; he had an agreement to teach at the University of California at Berkeley in 1983. Foucault died in Paris of an acquired immune-deficiency related illness.

HANS–GEORG GADAMER 1900–2002 CE

Born in Marburg, Germany, Gadamer was the son of a pharmacology professor and later university rector. Gadamer received his first doctoral degree at age 22 under the guidance of Plato scholar Paul Natorp. Gadamer was affected by polio a few months later; confined to his home, he read work by Husserl and Heidegger. He recovered, went to Freiburg to study with Heidegger, and became his assistant in 1923. Under Heidegger's direction, Gadamer received a second doctorate with a dissertation on Plato in 1928. He worked as a lecturer then as a professor teaching classical philosophy in Marburg. In 1939 he moved to the University of Leipzig; 7 years later, he becoming the university's rector. He returned to Frankfurt in 1947, where he became a professor in 1948; shortly thereafter, he occupied the professorial chair held by Karl Jaspers in Heidelberg until retiring in 1968. After retirement he was a visiting professor at numerous universities in the United States and internationally.

JÜRGEN HABERMAS 1929 CE –

Born in Düsseldorf, Habermas studied philosophy, history, psychology, and literature. He earned a Ph.D. degree in Bonn with a dissertation on the German Idealist Schelling. In 1956 he began work as a researcher at the Institute for Social Research (the Frankfurt School) and in 1964 became professor of sociology and philosophy in Frankfurt. From 1971 to 1981 he was the Director of the Max Planck Institute for Research into the Conditions of Life in the Scientific-Technical World. Later in his career he visited annually at Northwestern University in the United States.

CARL GUSTAV HEMPEL 1905–1997 CE

Born in Orianenburg, Germany, Hempel studied at the Realgymnasium in Berlin. He began his studies at the University of Gottingen in 1923, soon moved to the University of Heidelberg, then went to Berlin to study physics, math, and philosophy. Hempel met Reichenbach and members of the Berlin Circle while at Heidelberg. In 1929 he attended the first congress on scientific philosophy, which was organized by the Logical Positivists. He met Carnap at this congress; moved to Vienna; attended courses with Carnap, Schlick, and others; and attended meetings of the Vienna Circle. Hempel achieved the credentials necessary to teach at the secondary school level and earned a Ph.D. in 1934. Following completion of his doctorate, he emigrated to Belgium. In 1937 he received an invitation to join the University of Chicago as a research associate. He returned briefly to Belgium, then relocated to the United States in 1939 where he held positions at a number of prominent universities. He died in Princeton Township, New Jersey.

MARTIN HEIDEGGER 1889–1976 CE

Born in Messkirch, Baden, Germany, Heidegger studied theology early in his life in preparation for the priesthood. He worked closely with Husserl and dedicated his major work, *Being and Time,* to Husserl. He was appointed rector at the University of Freiburg but resigned this position. As a supporter of the National Socialist Movement in Germany, he was not allowed to teach again until 1951. There is a significant gap between his early and later works when he resumed publishing after returning to his career.

DAVID HUME 1711–1776 CE

Born in Edinburgh, Scotland, Hume spent most of his childhood in Chirnside, a village on the border of Scotland and England. He attended the University of Edinburgh for 3 years but did not complete a degree. He worked at a law firm when considering the study of law but did not find that a good fit. Hume began reading literature and philosophy extensively, suffered a nervous breakdown at age 18, recovered and worked in commerce briefly. He subsequently relocated to France where he wrote *A Treatise of Human Nature* (1739) followed by a lengthy history of Great Britain. Although his philosophy was well received in Scotland, his work gained little attention from others, with the exception of Kant, until the 20 century.

EDMUND HUSSERL 1859–1938 CE

Born in Moravia, Austria, Husserl was educated in Vienna and attended the University of Leipzig to work in physics and math. He later studied at the University of Berlin. Initially pursuing a realist approach in his work, he experienced considerable doubt in his own abilities as a philosopher and took a more Idealist direction with his work in phenomenology. Husserl held several academic positions at universities in Göttingen and Freiburg and named Heidegger successor to his position at the University of Freiburg. Because of Husserl's Jewish background, much of his work was smuggled out of Germany to avoid its destruction.

IMMANUEL KANT 1724–1804 CE

Born in Königsberg, East Prussia (now Kaliningrad, Russia), into a poor but strongly religious family, Kant is generally regarded as one of the most difficult to understand of all the philosophers. He was educated initially at a parochial school where he developed a distaste for organized religion. He attended the University of Königsberg at age 16 and graduated after 6 years. Unable to attain a teaching position, he worked as a tutor for affluent families. He returned to the University in 1755 and graduated with a doctoral degree with a dissertation focused on natural science. He became a lecturer in philosophy, mathematics, and natural science, and later a professor. He was known as a witty and engaging lecturer although his private life focused on reading and writing. Historians often report that his daily life was structured so rigidly that people would set their clocks by his daily walks.

THOMAS KUHN 1922–1996 CE

Born in Cincinnati, Ohio, United States, Kuhn received a Ph.D. in physics in 1949 from Harvard University. Kuhn was an assistant professor of the history of science at Harvard until 1956 when he began a position at the University of California-Berkeley. Kuhn became a full professor at Berkeley in 1961. In 1964, he accepted a position as M. Taylor Pyne Professor of Philosophy and History of Science at Princeton University where he remained until returning to Boston as a professor at Massachusetts Institute of Technology 1979. Kuhn received numerous prestigious awards and honorary degrees. He died of cancer in Cambridge, Massachusetts.

JOHN LOCKE 1632–1704 CE

Born in Wrington, Somerset, England, Locke had an early education that reflected the traditional scholastic and metaphysical focus of the times. Locke may have considered a career in the church but eventually pursued studies in medicine and natural philosophy. Locke was educated as a physician and studied under Robert Boyle, a prominent physicist at the time. Locke began his education at the University of Oxford in 1652 where he received early training in the classics and later in medicine and experimental science. Health problems and the political climate led to his relocation to France in 1675; he returned to England in 1679 then lived in the Netherlands during 1683 to 1688. He returned again to a more favorable political situation in England in 1689 and was later named Commissioner of Trade and Plantations, a position he held from 1696 to 1700 until retiring due to ill health.

STEPHEN TOULMIN 1922 CE –

Born in London, England, Toulmin earned an undergraduate degree in mathematics and physics from King's College in London and a Ph.D. from Cambridge in 1948. Toulmin had contact with Ludwig Wittgenstein at Cambridge and completed his dissertation as a Wittgensteinian analysis of ethics. Toulmin took a position initially as a lecturer in philosophy of science at Oxford and served as visiting professor in Australia. He later was a professor and chair of the department of philosophy at the University of Leeds and relocated to the United States in 1959 where he has held positions as a distinguished professor at numerous U.S. universities.

FOR FURTHER READING:

Aaron, R. I. (1971). *John Locke*. Clarendon Press.

Ackrill, J. L. (Ed.) (1981). *Aristotle the philosopher*. Oxford: Oxford University Press.

Craig, E. (1999). *Concise Routledge encyclopedia of philosophy*. London: Routledge.

Farrington, B. (1949). *Francis Bacon, philosopher of industrial science*. New York: H. Schuman.

Grene, M. (1998). *Descartes*. Indianapolis: Hackett Publishing Company.

Honderich, T. (1995). *Oxford companion to philosophy*. Oxford: Oxford University Press.

Inwood, M. (1997). *Heidegger*. Oxford: Oxford University Press.

Jolley, N. (1999). *Locke: His philosophical thought*. Oxford: Oxford University Press.

Kenny, A. (1993). *Descartes: A study of his philosophy*. St. Augustine.

Malpas, J., Arnswald, U., & Kertscher, J. (2002). *Gadamer's century*. Cambridge, MA: MIT Press.

O'Farrell, C. (1989). *Foucault: Historian or philosopher?* Macmillan.

Quinton, A. (1999). *Hume*. New York: Routledge.

Rasmussen, D., & Bernauer, J. (Eds) (1988). *The Final Foucault*. Cambridge, MA: MIT Press.

Scruton, R. (1983). *Kant*. Oxford: Oxford University Press.

Sharrock, W., & Read, R. (2002). *Kuhn: Philosopher of scientific revolution*. Malden, st MA: Blackwell Publishers.

Velarde-Mayol, V. (2000). *On Husserl*. Belmont, CA: Wadsworth Publishing.

Walker, R. C. S. (1999). *Kant*. New York: Routledge.

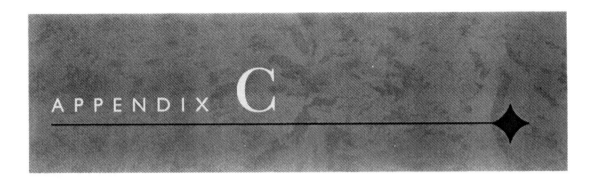

Selected Philosophy Internet Links

Individual philosophers and philosophical movements have their own followings. Google, Yahoo, or any of the Web search engines can provide more specific information on specific philosophers or philosophical traditions. The following are general starting points that may be a helpful adjunct to this text.

GENERAL PHILOSOPHY LINKS

Epipsteme Links: Electronic philosophy texts, philosopher info, and more
   http://www.epistemelinks.com/
Open Directory Project: Philosopher index
   http://dmoz.org/Society/Philosophy/Philosophers/
Internet Encyclopedia of Philosophy
   http://www.iep.utm.edu/
Stanford Encyclopedia of Philosophy
   http://plato.stanford.edu/contents-unabridged.html
World Wide Web Virtual Library: Philosophy
   http://www.bris.ac.uk/Depts/Philosophy/VL/
Erratic Impact Philosophy Research Database
   http://www.erraticimpact.com/
Internet History Sourcebook
   (has philosophy information as well particularly regarding science)
   http://www.fordham.edu/halsall/
Philosophy Pages
   http://www.philosophypages.com/hy/index.htm

TIMELINES

Timeline of Philosophy—Interactive
http://www.wadsworth.com/philosophy_d/special_features/timeline/timeline.html#
Radical Academy—Static timeline
http://radicalacademy.com/diahistphil.htm

ELECTRONIC TEXTS

Eserver—Electronic texts of all sorts including philosophy links
http://eserver.org/
The Internet Classics Archive
http://classics.mit.edu/
Kant's Critique of Pure Reason EText
http://www.arts.cuhk.edu.hk/Philosophy/Kant/cpr/
Institute for Learning Technologies, Columbia University
http://www.ilt.columbia.edu/publications/digitext.html

DICTIONARIES AND NOMENCLATURE

The Ism Book
http://www.saint-andre.com/ismbook/ism3.html
Philosophy Pages- dictionary
http://www.philosophypages.com/dy/index.htm

INDEX

Page numbers followed by f indicate figure; those followed by b indicate box; those followed by n indicate footnote

Breinigsville, PA USA
16 August 2010
243630BV00004B/2/A